D0202209

Chicken Soup for the Soul
Healthy Living:
Menopause

Jack Canfield

Mark Victor Hansen

Susan L. Hendrix, D.O.

PROFESSOR OF OBSTETRICS AND GYNECOLOGY
WAYNE STATE UNIVERSITY SCHOOL OF MEDICINE

Health Communications, Inc.
Deerfield Beach, Florida

www.hcibooks.com
www.chickensoup.com

We would like to acknowledge the many publishers and individuals who granted us permission to reprint the cited material.

Menopause Buddies reprinted by permission of Criss Bertling. ©2004 Criss Bertling.

Older Than the Shoemaker reprinted by permission of Marcia Byalick. ©2004 Marcia Byalick.

Passing the Baton reprinted by permission of Jenna Cassell. ©2004 Jenna Cassell.

(Continued on page 133)

Library of Congress Cataloging-in-Publication Data
is available from the Library of Congress

©2005 Jack Canfield and Mark Victor Hansen
ISBN 0-7573-0276-9

Publisher: Health Communications, Inc.
          3201 S.W. 15th Street
          Deerfield Beach, FL 33442–8190

Cover design by Larissa Hise Henoch
Inside book design by Lawna Patterson Oldfield
Inside book formatting Dawn Von Strolley Grove

Contents

Fear less, hope more,
eat less, chew more,
whine less, breathe more,
talk less, say more,
love more,
and all good things
will be yours.

—Swedish Proverb

Introduction: Menopause
Is a Time for Positive Changes

Today, women live half of their adult life after menopause. No longer is menopause the start of a slow decline into old age—rather, it's a fresh start, a liberating jump into new beginnings, with new possibilities and hope. You've reached a landmark time in your life, a goal worth celebrating.

But that doesn't mean it isn't a trying time as well. From health concerns to physical symptoms to simple fears of growing older, the pitfalls of menopause are real . . . but not nearly as bad as you've been led to believe.

There are many products today that claim to help women rid themselves of menopausal symptoms. It's up to you to educate yourself about what does and doesn't work. Read this book, talk to your doctor and be realistic. Menopause isn't something that can be cured—but many women do find relief from a combination of lifestyle changes. Some products do help some women, but it's important to remember that there is no magic bullet that will keep you young. I became well aware of this fact as one of the Principal Investigators of the Women's

Health Initiative, the study that found that hormone therapy can actually raise the risk of some deadly diseases.

What you need to do isn't easy and it isn't sexy—it's common sense. Eat a healthy diet, exercise regularly, and if you smoke, quit. These steps will help reduce many menopause symptoms and keep your body healthy as you begin the second half of your adult life. Make positive changes now—don't wait until you start feeling sick.

I get many questions from my patients about menopause. How long will menopause last? Should I take hormonal therapy? Is there hope for my sex life after menopause? What can I do about hot flashes? If I'm forgetful does that mean I'm starting to get Alzheimer's? These are all valid questions, and I'll answer them in the following pages. As you come up with questions of your own, I ask you to take the advice I give my patients: Ask your doctor, not your girlfriends. Every woman's experience with menopause is unique and can be a source of inspiration, as the essays in this book so vividly demonstrate. But what works for one woman won't necessarily work for someone else.

If you're a woman who is going through menopause or are about to, you've likely reached a point where you've experienced a range of life experiences that have given you a rich, deep perspective on life. Yes, you're going through changes, and some of them may be unpleasant, at least temporarily. But you're here, with many years ahead of you. If you have a meaningful, satisfying life, this is a wonderful time to reflect on all that you have and that you have accomplished. If you wish you could do more, be more, then this is the perfect time to act on your wishes.

I wish you luck and good health as you move through this tremendously important and life-changing journey.

Susan L. Hendrix, D.O.
Professor of Obstetrics and Gynecology
Wayne State University School of Medicine
Detroit, Michigan

My Menopause Journal

The ups, the downs, the opportunities, the challenges . . . there's so much going on when you're in menopause. Writing a menopause journal is a perfect way to capture those changes. It will help you sort through your physical changes and your thoughts about the future. It can help you work with your doctor, your spouse, your children, your friends and yourself. This book will feature numerous chances to add information to your menopause journal under the heading *Think About . . .*

You may want to treat yourself to a beautiful, leather-bound journal. Or you may be more comfortable typing your thoughts on a computer (but if you share the computer with family members, set up a password-protected area that only you can access). Or you may just want to scratch answers in the margins of this book. No matter your style, choose a regular time to write every day, and stick to it!

Eggs Over

My son, Graig, discovered Dr. Ruth when he was ten years old. He sat riveted to the television while I was preparing his favorite breakfast—French toast. As I was whipping up the eggs, I was half-listening as Dr. Ruth and a gynecologist were explaining menopause to the viewing audience. Suddenly, I was aware of a pair of eyes looking at me longingly. My son said nothing but continued to watch as I cooked. Finally, I asked if something was wrong. Wistfully, my son answered, "Did you know, Mommy, that after menopause, you can't make eggs anymore?"

♥ *Pat Gallant*

The Positive Side of Menopause

Menopause. It's a word loaded with associations—and usually not good ones. Hot flashes, mood swings, decreased sex drive, memory loss . . . these are the topics that are likely to pop up when you mention the "M" word. But menopause isn't a disease—it's a normal, healthy part of your life. In fact, it can be a time of liberation, change and innovation. A time to take up new interests, make healthful changes in your lifestyle, and strengthen relationships with loved ones. A time for new beginnings.

For many women, these are the years in which the children leave home. This means you can now invest more time in your career, explore hobbies you never had time for before, or go back to school. You can travel and spend more time with your spouse and friends. You can even have a romantic interlude with your husband again without your children interrupting!

Menopause is also a time to focus on your health, and this too can provide a wonderful opportunity to make changes in your lifestyle. If you haven't already started an exercise program and a healthy way of eating, now is certainly the time to do it—you'll feel better, and you'll protect yourself against many diseases of aging.

Don't forget that menopause isn't all about negative health changes. You'll no longer have to worry about PMS or unintended pregnancy—and for most of us, that's a very good thing!

Common Myths About Menopause . . . And Reasons Why You Should Question Them

Myth: Menopause is a uniformly awful experience, something to be dreaded.

Fact: Although women often do have some symptoms during menopause, there are ways to alleviate them. Many women find that menopause is a chance to focus more on themselves and make changes that will improve their health.

Myth: Forgetfulness is a common symptom of menopause.

Fact: Although you may feel as if you're constantly misplacing your keys or forgetting what you were about to do, in fact, there's no evidence that memory actually declines in women during menopause. Memory lapses during this time generally are caused by trying to do too many things at once. Menopause is not the best time for multitasking, especially with an infinite task list.

Myth: Depression is common in menopause.

Fact: While minor mood swings are common in menopause, depression is not a normal part of menopause. If you think you might be depressed, you should talk to your doctor, who can provide treatment if you are indeed found to be suffering from depression.

Myth: Gaining weight is inevitable during menopause.

Fact: With regular exercise and a healthy diet, you can prevent weight gain during menopause.

Myth: There aren't any alternatives to hormones to relieve menopause symptoms.

Fact: There are some botanical products and anti-depressants that may be helpful in relieving menopause symptoms. You can also make some lifestyle changes to help relieve symptoms. Besides, symptoms eventually go away, and with a positive attitude, they can be much more tolerable.

Myth: Once a woman starts skipping her period, she can't get pregnant.

Fact: You can still get pregnant even after you begin to miss periods. So unless you're trying to have a baby, be sure to use birth control until you haven't had any period for twelve months.

Passing the Baton

One is not born a woman, one becomes one.
—Simone De Beauvoir

Catherine casually looked in the mirror, then something caused her to linger. It was her mother looking back at her. She couldn't remember when her face had begun to age, wasn't aware of when the first line had appeared. Her plan had always been to age gracefully and naturally. Never to resort to coloring her hair in an attempt to appear different than she actually was, but to wear the gray like a badge of courage . . . like displaying a medal that was hard earned.

But she didn't plan for it to happen so soon. Didn't expect life to move so swiftly. How was it that, one minute at a time, the years had flown by her? Being older was always for other people. She expected it to come eventually, but it was supposed to come much, much later.

She needed a break from the image staring back at her with a shocked expression. She opened the medicine cabinet . . . giving her yet another image that, too, seemed to imitate her mother. The shelves were lined with medicine containers, each with her name neatly typed on it. There was no mistake as she checked the name on each vial . . . *Catherine Goodwin,* there like the salutation of a very personal letter.

One prescription at a time, she had filled the cabinet with this pill that increased her bone density, that pill that reduced the stiffness of her joints, another for a bout with situational depression, and yet one more to help when she couldn't sleep. Oddly enough, it was the smallest one of all that was the hardest to swallow . . . hormones.

Catherine had been forty-eight when she began experiencing pain in her abdomen. A gynecological exam and ultrasound revealed a uterus invaded by several large fibroid tumors. While she never had children, she'd imagined what it might be like to have something growing inside her. This was nothing like that.

She found herself facing a door that was wide open before her. The sign on the door said *Hysterectomy* and once a woman walked through, there was no turning back. It wasn't as if Catherine had planned to have children at this time in her life, she just didn't like the idea of being told she couldn't.

She was in limbo. After a twenty-five-year marriage—a quarter of a century—her husband
turned their lives into a caricature of a midlife
couple by leaving her for another woman. She was
standing at the doorway of losing her feminine
organs and facing it alone. Then, to make matters
worse, a fire welled up from inside and burned out
from every pore in what felt like a personal visit to
hell. "Hot flash" seemed too mild a term to describe
it, as it was hotter than hot and lasted a lot longer
than a flash.

Catherine wasn't the type of person to wallow in
self-pity. She was a woman of action. Rather than
trust the medical community, she decided to
approach every elderly woman she came across. She
was looking for the sage advice of those who had
actually been through it or were also walking the path
beyond the door of menopause—to share the journey into this challenging transitional phase of life.

She conducted her research everywhere she
went. Whether in the park, at a restaurant, in a
movie theater or at the gym, she found pre-
menopausal, perimenopausal, menopausal and
postmenopausal women eager to share experiences.

In the gym locker room, an eighty-year-old
woman stood naked, in all her proud feminine
glory and smiled knowingly. "It will be alright,
honey," she said kindly. "You are still young and

have a lot more to experience long after the change." Catherine realized she had been feeling too old to be "young," but too young to be "old." It was nice to put things into long-term perspective and to just be in the presence of such grace.

In response to her questions, a group of fifty-something women on a picnic in the park were laughing and singing, "We love our hysterectomies!" They reminded Catherine that along with the ability to reproduce, one loses a very large monthly inconvenience. This same group suggested that instead of cursing the discomfort while in the midst of a hot flash, to instead be glad for the sudden power surge!

Catherine decided to go ahead with the surgery and was able to have a vaginal hysterectomy so the recovery was less traumatic. She wouldn't have known this was an option if she hadn't "researched" it—none of her doctors had suggested this option.

The first time she went to the drugstore after the surgery, she stood in front of the tampon display and cried. It wasn't that she would miss using them; it was more of what it represented. When she found a lone tampon in her gym bag, she cried again and couldn't bring herself to remove it.

That afternoon, while back in the gym locker room, a panicked voice came from the bathroom. "Oh, no!! Does anyone have a tampon?" Catherine smiled and reached into her bag. She walked into the bathroom area and found a young, redheaded woman looking around frantically. As Catherine handed her the tampon, she felt as if she were passing the baton at an Olympic event. This young woman was her team member, and it was her turn to run.

♥ *Jenna Cassell*

What Is Menopause?

Menopause is not a sudden event. It is a normal, natural and slowly evolving part of a woman's life. Your body's level of the hormone estrogen falls to very low levels, and your menstrual periods stop. You are officially considered to be going through menopause when you haven't had a period for twelve months in a row, if other causes have been ruled out.

Menopause usually begins between the ages of forty-five to fifty-five, with the average age being fifty-one. There is a wide range, however—in rare cases, women reach natural menopause as early as their thirties (called premature menopause) or as late as their sixties. Smoking can speed up menopause by one to two years. Surgery to remove ovaries also causes menopause.

Before natural menopause begins, you go through a phase called **perimenopause**. You may have intense symptoms such as hot flashes and mood swings, and you may have changes in your period. The good news is that menopause brings relief from regular periods and cramps.

Luckily, there are many steps you can take to alleviate your symptoms—through eating changes, exercise, stress reduction techniques, medication and nondrug alternatives. We'll explore your choices in the following chapters. The important thing is to listen to your body, observe the changes closely, and work with your health care provider to keep your body strong and comfortable as you go through this life-changing time.

🌀 Think about . . .
my attitude toward menopause

My positive thoughts about menopause are:

_____

_____

My biggest fears about menopause are:

_____

_____

Five ways my life will improve after menopause
are:

_____

_____

My goals for menopause are:

_____

_____

My goals for life after menopause are:

_____

_____

HRT (Husband Response Therapy)

H oney,

First of all, this is not a "Dear John" letter, as you may have thought. Things aren't that bad. It's a note to try to help you understand what I'm going through. I'm sure if I tried to discuss this with you in person, you'd be backing your way out of the house, slinking into the sanctuary that is your garage, as I went on and on. So I'm putting it in writing. Go get yourself a cup of coffee, a cold beer—whatever—but please read this.

I don't know where to start. All of a sudden it's as if I'm no longer in control of my body. I'm gaining weight. I'm tired all the time. I'm easily annoyed (I guess you know that) and it seems as if I have no interest in sex—but then you were the first to figure that one out, too. At first I thought I was crazy, that I was losing my mind! Then I began to talk to my friends about my symptoms and discovered they're all feeling the same way. It's safe to say, so are their husbands. Most of our mothers never discussed "the change" with us. Their generation avoided the subject, so in many ways this is all new to us.

I've discovered, oddly enough, that this is all normal for women my age: the hot flashes, the anxiety, the irregular periods . . . I could go on, but I'm sure you don't want all the details. All you need to know is that you're not really married to a nutcase. I'm normal.

On top of all these horrible symptoms, there's so much confusion over what to do about them. I could take hormones and get rid of most of them, but then I may be exposing myself to an increased risk of breast cancer, heart disease, dementia . . . that list goes on and on, according to the Women's Health Initiative study. So I'm not sure what to do. I want to get help but I'm afraid of the long-term consequences.

Whatever I decide, know that I want you by my side, even if as I say that, I'm pushing you away. When I snap at you for saying something I would have laughed at a few days ago, I silently ask myself how I could be so thoughtless but I can't seem to get past the anger to apologize. For those times, I'm saying it now. I'm sorry.

I don't expect you to read all the books I'm reading. I don't really want you to come to my doctor visits. I just want you to tell me that you still love me, to put your arms around me every now and then, to pamper me just a little, and to stay the heck away when you can tell I'm about to explode. That's all.

I've been reading a lot lately and I've found that more than half of women who are postmenopausal feel that they are the happiest they've been in their entire lives. Hold that thought, we'll get there.

Love,

Me

♥ *Kimberly Porrazzo*

Menopause Buddies

You're dying for a caffeine fix because you have the energy level of a woman who's just given birth after twenty-four hours of hard labor. But experience has taught you that within a mere 120 seconds of sipping that cup of Komodo Dragon Bold Java, you'll feel like you've been buried in an anthill and dowsed with boiling water. So you drink water—again. Of course, you've learned to be in close proximity to a ladies' room shortly after gulping down that 32 ounces of natural spring nectar.

Call your Menopause Buddy.

Your gravity-challenged body becomes home to creeping cellulite deposits. You need glasses to read the carbohydrate and fat grams on those Barbie-size boxes of frozen diet meals. You begin to sleep on the side of the bed closest to the bathroom because you're spending a lot of time getting up in the middle of the night to go there. You have to change the bed sheets frequently because of some-thing called "night sweats."

Call your Menopause Buddy.

Mental-pause is a strange brain disorder that occurs during this season of life. You are forever asking yourself questions like: Why did I get out of my chair? Was I supposed to call someone? Why am I staring at that computer screen, was I doing something important? What is my firstborn's name?

Call your Menopause Buddy.

My best friend and I have been on the Menopause Buddy System for about ten years now. When we were both age forty-five, she would say things to me like, "Honey, you look awful. I just don't know how that feels." She never had hot sweats, she still got up at 5 a.m. to work out three mornings a week, and she didn't have beastly mood swings.

"I'm so blessed," she would offer. "My mother never had symptoms either. But I know you must feel just terrible." *Lucky me,* I thought. My mother turned into the Wicked Witch of the West during menopause and passed that legacy down to me. Even the mailman was begging me to go on hormone replacement therapy!

There is nothing like a Menopause Buddy during the years when the young you begins to fade and your mother is the person you see when you look in the mirror.

Your Menopause Buddy thinks it's hysterical when you have made plans to meet for lunch and you go to one restaurant while she goes to another. She loves swapping mental-pause stories about putting the ice cream in the dishwasher or discovering the Tide in the refrigerator.

Your Menopause Buddy empathizes when you feel yourself disappear and wonder if you're ever coming back. She forgives you when your words are short or even unkind because your hormone levels are off. She's the first one to laugh with you and the first one to comfort you.

During my menopausal years I have lost both of my parents and my husband. My Menopause Buddy has lost her parents and a dear friend. I have been blessed with two grandchildren. She has been blessed with three. Both of us have lost jobs, changed careers, and had financial ups and downs.

An entire decade has passed and my Menopause Buddy and I are still dealing with symptoms and issues. We wonder when it will finally end. We have decided, however, that we like being in some stage of menopause because it means we're not yet officially senior citizens.

We still compare notes. We still cry together and laugh even more. Our children still think we're a little nuts. But giggling with your best friend through the torrential sweats of a hot flash makes menopause a time of treasured memories.

♥ *Criss Bertling*

Talk About Menopause

Menopause is a personal journey, and you may not necessarily feel like sharing your every mood and hot flash with family and friends. But it's important that the people around you know that you are going through changes—for your sake *and* theirs. Be sure to talk about changes to:

- Your mood
- Your sleep
- Your ability to concentrate
- Your anxiety level
- Anything else you are experiencing

It's important to realize that all women experience menopause differently. Every woman's body is unique. Just because your mother or your sister or your best friend had certain symptoms at this time of her life, it doesn't mean that you will. If you have questions about menopause, be sure to ask your doctor—he or she will have access to the latest information on the best ways to deal with the changes you're going through.

Keep Communication Lines Open

It won't do you or anyone else around you any good to hide your feelings and changes as you go through menopause. If you're feeling irritable, tired and generally hormonal, warn those around you, and ask them in advance for their understanding. Try these strategies:

- I will ask my spouse to spend more time with our children if I feel my stress levels are interfering with open and constructive communication with them.
- I'll discuss the changes I'm experiencing at a time when I'm feeling good, not during a hormonal outburst.
- I'll ask my spouse to try to have patience as I make my way through this new time in my life.
- I'll use this opportunity to talk about trying out new ways of intimacy. I'll work on telling my partner what I think is exciting and desirable, and find out my partner's wishes and desires, too.

Keep Your Partner Involved

You have a lot of choices to make during menopause. Yes, the ultimate decisions are up to you, but keeping your partner involved along the way can improve communication between you. Good ways of involving your partner include discussing the pros and cons of hormone therapy, and jointly developing a plan to eat better and exercise more.

Talking to Your Kids

If your children are teenagers, then mood swings are rampant throughout the house! Having a talk with your teenage kids about what you're going through during menopause may seem like quite a challenge, but it can really pay off in terms of family peace!

When talking to your teens

- Make the connection between your hormonal changes and theirs.
- Be sure to explain that you're not sick— menopause is a natural process that all women go through.
- Ask your kids to help you—for instance, by instituting an hour of quiet in the house every evening or by taking a daily walk with you.

🕸 *Think about . . .*
talking about menopause

The time and place I feel most comfortable talking about menopause with my husband is:

_____

_____

The time and place I feel most comfortable talking about menopause with my children is:

_____

_____

The time and place I feel most comfortable talking about menopause with my friends is:

_____

_____

The person I feel most comfortable talking about menopause with is:

_____

_____

When I am feeling bad, I will:

_____

_____

_____

When I am feeling good, I will:

_____

_____

_____

When I talk to people I trust about menopause, here's what I will ask them to do to help me:

_____

_____

_____

Now that you have your answers, plan specific times within the next two weeks to talk about what you're experiencing. It's great for them— but it will be even better for you!

_____

_____

_____

Male Menopause

Remember, you may not be the only one in your household experiencing hormone changes. If you have teenagers in the house, you know what I mean. And your spouse may be going through "male menopause," producing less of the male hormone testosterone just as you're producing less estrogen. Some common symptoms of male menopause sound familiar—hot flashes, sleep problems, mood swings and decreased sexual desire.

If you are indeed going through hormonal changes at the same time as your spouse, have some sympathy for him—while women expect to go through menopause, men don't. And men aren't as likely to feel comfortable talking about their physical and emotional changes: Unless your spouse is unusually in touch with his feelings, he's unlikely to want to admit, much less discuss, what he's going through. That means it's up to you to be the family's main communicator—but aren't you already?

Turning Up the Heat

We boil at different degrees.

—RALPH WALDO EMERSON

It probably should have dawned on me that menopause was finally knocking on my door the day my husband muttered, through oddly chattering teeth, "Think we need to push the thermostat just a touch higher, Hon?" I had to stop for a moment and ponder this, savoring the sudden turnaround.

"Let me get this straight," I countered, lifting my sleeveless top just a little to fan myself. "After all these years of heating bill wars, now you're the one who's cold? It's like a sauna in here, John." I rearranged my hair atop my head, in a knot. Even my neck was sweating.

Part way through what I immediately seized as a splendid opportunity to razz my spouse about his aging process—as in, "I hear the older you get, the colder you get . . . ," my out-of-the-nest-but-never-too-far-from-free-laundry-facilities son, Chris, stomped his way into my kitchen, bringing a blast of frigid wind and a trail of slush with him. He plopped his groaning basket of dirty clothes on the table, yanking off his gloves with his teeth. "It's miserable out there. A little chilly in here, too."

John stood there in his thick Irish knit sweater, arms folded smugly across his chest. "Yup. That's what I said. Your mother is hot."

"Oh, it's probably that female thing." Chris had just enough time to scoot past me and jack up the heat before I nailed him squarely on the back of his head with his own box of dryer sheets.

I sank into the ladder-back chair, the one that seemed to be squeaking a little more loudly lately, and was becoming just a tad uncomfortable. Its caned seat felt scratchy against the back of my legs. There I sat, still feeling for the life of me like the whole house was a steam room, clad in a tank top and the shortest shorts I could find and would no longer dare to wear in public. The two men in my life looked as if they belonged in another climate altogether. John was bundled up and looked ready to pose for the annual Christmas card. Chris was still in his parka, blowing warm breath onto his hands and checking to see if the thermometer was rising.

"Gonna throw these in. I bet it's nice and warm by the dryer!" Chris grabbed his laundry basket, elbowing his father on the way. The two of them were chuckling as they headed down the hall. Suddenly, I hated men.

A female thing. That's what my only boy-child—the one I'd made sure knew how to do his own laundry, cook his own dinner, and by golly, never make distinctions as to what women can and cannot do—said to me, his mother. And his father—who'd applauded loudly when, back when we were young, I'd broken through the glass ceiling at work and garnered "a man's job"—laughing along with him? Now, my husband changed into Mr. Condescending to the Little Woman? Who were these two, anyway? I wasn't feeling so much overheated now as I was angry and a little bit weepy.

My legs began itching again, and I headed for the lotion bottle. It was getting low again. *Someone must be drinking this stuff,* I thought. I kicked off the shorts and yanked on my good old reliable sweatpants, the ones that don't care when I have fat days. And then, though I hated to admit it, I was beginning to feel cold. Itchy, but cold.

"You know, Dad, that's what it has to be." I could hear Chris speaking, barely audible. "Yeah, I know it, and you know it," John whispered. "And she knows it, too. Give it time."

If I'd heard that a half an hour earlier, I probably would have ridden into the laundry room on my broomstick and given them a talking to, judging that discussion behind my back uncalled for. Instead, I lit a couple of jasmine-scented candles, turned out the bathroom light and sat in a steamy tub until the water nearly turned cold. The flickering light cast forgiving shadows on my naked body, smoothing over the wrinkles that were not there yesterday.

John knocked on the door. "You okay in there?"

"Yeah. Come on in." I stretched to grab a towel, to cover up even though my long-suffering husband knew every imperfect inch. He reached for it instead and knelt by the tub, looking very young in the candlelight. He kissed me and wrapped the towel around my shoulders, and for just a moment, nothing itched, ached or felt bloated. "Turn up the heat," I murmured.

"Wouldn't have it any other way." He smiled. I felt warm again, but it wasn't a hot flash. I know the difference now. Some things can't be controlled: the weather, the passage of time, the hormonal rush. Or, for that matter, the fire inside.

♥ *Candy Killion*

The ABCs of Menopause

A   Always take time for yourself
B   Be flexible
C   Cut yourself some slack
D   Do something new
E   Enjoy each moment
F   Find a hobby
G   Get a new outfit
H   Hug everyone around you
I   Ideas are everywhere
J   Join a support group
K   Keep a sense of humor
L   Let go of small disagreements
M   Make a date with a loved one once a month
N   Notice the birds singing
O   Open a journal and write
P   Put together a memory box
Q   Quit thinking negatively
R   Remember to thank those who've supported you
S   Support a new charity
T   Take a walk with someone
U   Use a special talent to surprise a friend

V   Voice your opinions with truth and love
W   Wishes come true
X   Extra patience will pay off
Y   You are important and don't you forget it!
Z   Plenty of zzzzzz's will calm emotions and your
    heart

♥ *Deborah Bates Cavitt*

Relieve Your Symptoms

Hot Flashes

Hot flashes are the symptoms most commonly associated with menopause. They are most likely to occur in the year or two just before and after your period stops. Hot flashes are a sudden feeling of heat mostly in the upper part of your body. Your face and neck become flushed, and you may see red blotches on your chest, back and arms. The hot flash can be followed by heavy sweating and cold shivering. Some women who get hot flashes describe it as a light blush, while others have severe nighttime flashes that wake them up from a sound sleep, called **night sweats**. Flashes usually last between thirty seconds and five minutes. Hot flashes can occur anywhere from once a month to several times an hour.

Lifestyle Changes

Learning to overcome your hot flashes is a very empowering feeling. Try these lifestyle changes to help with hot flashes:

- Dress in layers so you can remove some of your clothing when you feel warm. (Those old turtlenecks may have to go!)

- Sleep in a cool room.
- If you have night sweats, wear a short, cool cotton nightshirt to bed and have an extra set nearby. Some women do best sleeping with nothing on under a cotton sheet. Keep a glass of ice water next to the bed.
- Identify hot flash triggers such as hot spicy foods, alcohol and beverages.
- Reduce caffeine.
- Meditate or do yoga or relaxation exercises.
- Exercise. Some women find that regular exercise brings relief from hot flashes and other symptoms.
- If you feel a hot flash coming on, sip a cool drink.

Paced breathing

Paced breathing helps some women control hot flashes. Here's how you do it:

- Find a quiet, comfortable place to sit where you won't be distracted.
- Breathe from deep inside your abdomen while slowing your breaths to five or six times a minute (we normally breathe ten to fifteen times a minute).
- Practice breathing in for five seconds and breathing out for five seconds to get the correct timing.
- Do this for fifteen minutes a day.

• When you feel a hot flash coming on, try decreasing your breathing to help stop the hot flash cold.

Sleep Problems

There are many reasons why you may have problems sleeping. Mostly, it's from waking up because of night sweats—but anxiety can also play a role.

Good sleep, which is so important for your physical and mental well-being, is especially important because you need to be well-rested to cope with the challenges you may face as you go through menopause.

Some simple ways to improve your sleep include:

• Doing physical activity in the morning or early afternoon—exercising later in the day may increase wakefulness at night.

• Taking a hot shower or bath immediately before going to bed.

• Avoiding alcohol, caffeine, larger meals and working right before bedtime.

• Try drinking herb tea or warm milk before bed.

• Keeping your bedroom at a comfortable temperature.

• Avoiding napping during the day. Try to get to bed and get up on a regular schedule.

• Using light-blocking window shades or wearing a sleep mask.

• Closing doors and windows to block out sound.

Memory Problems

Forgetfulness and fuzzy brain are common complaints during menopause. But menopause itself doesn't cause memory problems; for most women, problems with concentrating and not remembering where they put things stem from too many worries and concerns.

There are some commonsense ways to de-stress your body, including getting enough sleep, staying physically active and eating a healthy diet. In addition, try some relaxation exercises to keep you centered.

Here's a relaxation exercise to do once a day:

1. Sit quietly in a comfortable position and close your eyes.
2. Deeply relax all your muscles.
3. Breathe in and out through your nose, silently repeating a word or phrase.
4. Continue for ten to twenty minutes.
5. Slowly open your eyes and return to full consciousness.

Involuntary Urine Release

Stress urinary incontinence happens when urine leaks when you sneeze, laugh, cough or exercise. Don't worry, it's normal, although being overweight does increase the risk. Here's an easy exercise, called a Kegel exercise, that will strengthen the muscle that allows you to keep the urine from leaking out unexpectedly.

To locate the muscle, try stopping and starting the flow of urine. When you feel it, simply tighten and relax the muscle over and over, about twenty times, three times a day.

Overactive Bladder

An overactive bladder causes you to feel that you must urinate more frequently than usual, or you will get a sudden strong need to urinate immediately. Perhaps most distressing is the leakage of urine that follows a sudden, strong urge. If you have an overactive bladder, see your doctor—he or she may prescribe medication to help.

Some medicines, such as high blood pressure drugs, may increase your output of urine and can lead to an overactive bladder. Ask your doctor if taking a different kind of medicine may solve the problem.

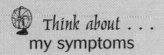
Think about . . .
my symptoms

Rate the following symptoms on a scale of 1 to 10, 10 being the most serious, then note your current treatments. Bring the list to your next doctor's visit to help figure out your best options.

_____ Hot flashes

_____ Mood swings

_____ Trouble sleeping

_____ Memory or concentration problems

_____ Needing to suddenly go to the bathroom

_____ Decreased sex drive

_____ Vaginal dryness

Here's what I've used to treat menopause symptoms, and how well they worked:

Treatment	Very Effective	Somewhat Effective	Not Effective
1.			
2.			
3.			
4.			
5.			
6.			
7.			
8.			
9.			

Wanted: One Inner Crone

Having stumbled my way into menstruation at the tender age of eleven, I had hoped to march into an early menopause. I figured twenty-five, thirty years tops, from start to finish. No such luck.

After almost forty years of checking the calendar, not to mention my underwear, on a monthly basis, I've had it. I'm more than ready to cast off the moon goddess and her cyclical visitations of fertility, and embrace my inner crone.

Instead of obsessing about mundane things like lipstick shades, the numbers on the bathroom scale and what to make for dinner, I will be transformed into a wise and caring Earth goddess. I will shower the world with love and understanding. I will be one with nature. Not having to deal with monthly bloating and cravings would also be nice.

Unfortunately, my recalcitrant crone is not ready to embrace me back.

A few times over the last two years, she's danced into my life, only to glide out again three months later, leaving me once more to reach into the medicine cabinet for a tampon and circle another date on the calendar. I remain stranded in the purgatory of perimenopause, while my friends continue their journey into wisdom without me.

I've read dozens of books on menopause. I've increased my intake of soy to make the transition easier. I've even allowed the gray hairs to inch, okay gallop, their way forward. What more does my tardy crone want?

In the meantime, she teases me with symptoms. Hot flashes ripple through my body and leave me breathless and sweating—with no gorgeous hunk in sight.

Lust I could handle. A malfunctioning internal thermometer renders me ridiculous, a radiator with no off button. I stand in front of the open refrigerator, waiting for its cooling breeze to return my body to some sense of normalcy, as I idly nibble on whatever leftovers have not evolved into new life forms.

Mood swings make getting up in the morning an adventure. I never know which of me will climb out of bed—the good twin or the evil twin. My family and longtime friends point out that my middle name was always "moody," but I think they're just jealous that I have a built-in excuse for being miserable.

As a career cynic, I'm embarrassed to find myself

crying at corny commercials or maudlin Hallmark cards.

My prankster crone taunts me with meno-"pauses," irritating lapses in memory that strike without rhyme or reason. I walk out of a room intent on retrieving an item, and a minute later I am reduced to wondering what I wanted. I prowl around the house, hoping the sight of something will trigger my memory. It doesn't.

Desperate, I bought a book on how to improve my memory, but my crafty crone descended long enough to hide the book. It's probably next to my missing ginkgo biloba pills, billed as an ancient Chinese memory enhancer—but only if you can find them.

Even if I could remember what I wanted, I probably couldn't find the right word for it. Yes, I am slowly losing my nouns, stolen no doubt by my tight-lipped crone. I am reduced to describing common objects as thingamajigs or whatcha-macallits or doohickeys. Pointing to objects in my own house is frustrating, but when I have to do it at work, it's humiliating.

Darn it, I'm an English as a Second Language teacher and freelance writer. Words were my specialty. Now they're my nemesis. Luckily, my students are used to fumbling for words in English, and they sit patiently while I struggle to dredge up the right expression. And several other teachers are in the same thingamajig I'm in. That doohickey that floats on water. Boat, they're in the same boat I'm in. So they nod sympathetically when I flounder.

Editors aren't quite as understanding. I find myself writing articles and putting X's in places where I can't think of the term I want. Soon the X's will outnumber the actual words.

As I sit on the couch, sobbing over some stupid made-for-TV movie, a chocolate bar in one hand and a XXXXXXXX (to be filled in later, I hope) in the other, I wonder what else I can do to entice my treacherous crone. Buy a nicer couch? Eat imported chocolate? Install a satellite dish so I can watch better movies?

If my inner crone doesn't show up soon and turn me into a wise, compassionate and loving woman, I'm going to wring her wrinkled little neck.

♥ *Harriet Cooper*

Mentalpause: ('men-tel poz /)

N **oun:** The period of natural cessation of mental clarity, aggravated by age, hormones, including, but not limited to, such thought-provoking subjects as: the price, need, availability and significance of paper products.

Verb: The act of whizzing past the diaper aisle without a second thought or a tinge of baby lust, then cruising past the feminine protection department, pausing . . .

1. And in the blink of a bifocaled eye realizing that the next "lane" consists mainly of bladder control products.
2. Experiencing a sudden philosophical hot flash (aka power surge) of perspiration-induced inspiration while simultaneously realizing that a woman's entire life cycle can be summarized in three grocery aisles.
3. Deciding not to get panty hose in a cold sweat over it all and continuing on to "apparel" and commencing to fill aforementioned cart with trendy clothing and a few new rap CDs.

4. Then wondering, while leaving the store . . .
5. Now where did I park the car?

Adjective: *Mentalpausaly:* Having achieved a state of higher cognitive processing capabilities, while intermittently experiencing technical difficulties.

Adverb: *Mentalpausal:* Of, relating to or describing certain mature, womanly phenomena.

♥ *Jacqueline J. Michels*

Mood Swings

Mood swings are a hallmark of menopause. You may feel irritable, on edge, and just "not yourself." Or you may quickly go from feelings of elation to a quick flash of anger. Things that might not have bothered you in the past may now cause you to blow up suddenly. That unpredictability can be pretty unsettling to you, and to those around you.

Hormone changes are certainly one reason your mood may shift suddenly throughout the day. Other causes include your reaction to hot flashes and fatigue due to poor sleep. Add all that to the stressful life changes that you may be experiencing as you face growing older, your children leave home and your parents' health starts declining, and it's no wonder you're moody!

Dealing with Mood Swings

Mood swings are a normal part of the menopause years. Don't feel guilty about them! But don't let them control you, either. You can

- Tell those around you—family, coworkers and friends—to let you know (when your mood is good) when you may seem on edge more than in the past.

- Give loved ones permission to talk about how your mood swings are affecting their relationship with you.
- Take a deep breath and think before saying what you really think in a moment of anger—remember, you can't take it back!

🌀 Think about . . .
what causes my stress

To find out what causes you the most stress, make a three-column list. In the first column, list your causes of stress (such as not having enough time, your kids or your finances). In the second column, list how your body and emotions react to stress (such as your heart pumping quickly or your neck muscles hurting). In the third column, list what you do when you get stressed (such as yelling, running to the fridge or smoking).

Take a close look at your answers. What do you have control over? Are your warning signs dangerous to your health? Are your responses to stress healthy or not?

If you're like many women, much of your stress comes from simply trying to do too much. How do you really spend your time? Create a pie chart and find out. Draw a circle and divide it into pie slices according to your many activities. Include work, taking care of the house and children, sleeping, watching TV, talking on the phone, driving and cooking. In each slice, write down the activity and about how long you spend on it every day. Make bigger slices for the activities that you spend the most time doing.

Now take a look at the pie. Are you spending most of your time doing things that create stress? Are there any activities you could increase or decrease to reduce your stress level? Is there enough fun in your daily pie?

Depression Isn't Normal

While mood swings may be normal during menopause, depression isn't. Depression can be debilitating, limiting your daily activities. Women at greatest risk of depression are those who have a history of depression, including depression after childbirth (postpartum) and women who have felt depressed around the time of their menstrual periods.

It's important to know that depression is a treatable medical illness. If you experience any of the following for more than two weeks, see your doctor.

- An "empty" feeling, ongoing sadness and anxiety
- Tiredness, lack of energy
- Loss of interest or pleasure in everyday activities, including sex

- Sleep problems, including trouble getting to sleep, very early morning waking and sleeping too much
- Eating more or less than usual
- Crying too often or too much
- Aches and pains that don't go away when treated
- A hard time focusing, remembering or making decisions
- Feeling guilty, helpless, worthless or hopeless
- Being irritable
- Thoughts of death or suicide

My Page

My Thoughts _____
_____
_____
_____

My Feelings _____
_____
_____
_____

My Facts _____
_____
_____
_____

My Support _____
_____
_____
_____

Older Than the Shoemaker

I was sold a bill of goods. The same people who advised me to curtail my outdoor activities the summer of my thirteenth year so I wouldn't embarrass myself by "gushing blood" all over my white pants, who warned me adolescence was going to be five years of pimples, mood swings and broken hearts, who told me childbirth felt like pulling your top lip up over your forehead . . . these prophets of doom and gloom swore menopause was the most miserable time of all.

They of the furrowed brow and downturned mouth sighed about the awful inevitability of becoming invisible to the opposite sex. The entire geography of my body would soon lower a good six inches, they forecast, melting into rolls of prune-like wrinkled flesh. There would be no escaping this ghastly fate.

I bought their tales as a budding teenager, but as a blooming menopausal woman, I know their sour words reveal more about their temperament than any truth. What physical symptoms I've experienced are more irritating than life-altering. And in return for these minor annoyances comes a clear, brilliant consciousness. For the first time I recognize my responsibility in my own health care. I am aware that what I eat and how I sleep and how I commit to exercise will determine how I look and feel . . . and how I handle menopause. No longer dwelling on the externals, I accept my body as a walking autobiography of the major and minor stresses of my life. Rather than sliding downhill, I'm struggling up steep mountains I was too timid and shy to attempt earlier. Since my periods ended, I began a new career, took up spinning (a challenging indoor cycling regimen), gave myself permission to end two unsatisfactory friendships, mastered the computer, became closer to becoming the mother I always tried to be and fell in love with my husband all over again. I'm not revised or refreshed or reconfigured . . . I'm all new.

As a younger woman, my behavior was determined by the plans other people had in mind. My generation adhered strictly to the rules—graduation, marriage, kids—I was finished with all I was supposed to do by thirty. Today I am more concentrated, more radical, more clearly myself than I was in the revolutionary sixties when I worried about whether my lipstick was white enough. Now that I'm older than my shoemaker (he's fifty-two!), challenges no longer frighten me; they tap reserves of confidence I never knew I possessed. During menopause I've explored the option of just letting things happen, not easy for a control freak. In return, I've learned to breathe, to balance, to trust that the world will not end if I am not in charge.

Anna Quindlen once said a finished person is a boring person. At this time of my life, I exult in feeling less "finished" than ever before. I look back at the long, other-directed years of my youth as worth living precisely because I've arrived here now. I'm enjoying the sunny afternoon of my life and have no desire to prolong the morning. At this moment I'm not interested in hitting the delete key to remove my wrinkles with plastic surgery. Turning back towards youth or treading water to remain stationary seems a foolish expenditure of energy. After all, it took fifty years to feel this optimistic and I don't want to waste a moment of this precious time.

♥ *Marcia Byalick*

Lessen the Stress

With so many physical and emotional changes going on, it's no wonder you probably feel stressed out! You can—and should—sit down and take inventory of everything that's going on in your life and decide what changes you can make to lessen the stress level. In addition to eating right, exercising and creating relaxing sleep rituals, here are some ideas:

Get support. You may be feeling overwhelmed—in addition to your own midlife changes, you may be caring for children as well as elderly parents. Don't be shy about asking for help from your spouse, friends or relatives if you find you can't handle all your responsibilities at once.

Get professional help. If you're helping your aging parents, see if there are community resources that can help with some of the responsibilities, such as a meal delivery service or a visiting nurse.

Work with your boss. Would a more flexible schedule make life easier for you? If you've been at your job for awhile, your boss may be willing to work with you to make your hours more manageable—perhaps you can get in earlier and leave earlier to avoid rush-hour traffic, for instance.

Spend time with others. Women who are stressed

tend to withdraw from others, thinking that they're not good company. But being around other people is important. If you live alone, consider joining a support group.

Find time for activities you enjoy. You may not feel like doing much of anything, but avoiding your old favorite activities is likely to just make you feel worse. Keep on doing things you used to like to do, and you'll find you start enjoying yourself again, even if it's only for short periods at first.

Try yoga. Relaxation techniques such as yoga or tai chi can help even out the emotional ups and downs of menopause.

Chase away negative thoughts about yourself. Yes, we're all guilty of it being quick to list our faults. Pick a time when you're in a positive frame of mind. Then go ahead—write down those negative thoughts, followed by specific examples of why they're not true. For instance, if you write down that you've been short-tempered with everyone, think about that time you spent hours on the phone with a friend in need.

Make a list of your best qualities. If the changes you're going through are getting you down, now's a great time to remember what makes you so special. Yes, ideally your family and friends remind you, but let's be realistic! Take time to appreciate your strengths—and write them down so you can refer to them when you're feeling low.

Be kind to yourself. Menopause is a time of major changes, so it's not unusual for you to not always feel like your old self. You're finding a way to your new self, so give it time.

🌐 *Think about . . .*
how to lessen my stress

When I feel stressed out I can

1._____

2._____

3._____

4._____

5._____

Sometimes I think this negative thing about myself:

_____

_____

But here's why it's not true:

_____

_____

My best qualities are:

_____

_____

Stopping and Starting

Women complain about sex more often than men.
Their gripes fall into two major categories:
(1) Not enough. (2) Too much.

—ANN LANDERS

Go figure. You still feel like a young girl just home from the prom, but suddenly your girlfriends are whispering, "Have you stopped?" instead of "Have you started?"

And then your granddaughter confesses she's started, and you realize your prom corsage is, well, wilted. Just like you feel.

I was crabby. Flushing. Up and down emotionally. An early hysterectomy had left me my ovaries but not the most notable sign of menopause. I'd "stopped" two decades earlier.

Unsure, I turned to my funny friend Glennis, a few rungs higher on the ladder to eternity. Was irritability a sure sign of menopause?

"Irritability?" she repeated. "Well, a few years back, my husband, George, developed a very irritating habit. He'd breathe in. Then a few seconds later, he'd breathe out. And he kept *doing* it!"

Well, I wasn't alone. I had to do something. The women's magazines urged me toward synthetic hormones. My son the herbalist promised plants could dispel my hot flashes, my moods, and—well, all those people who kept breathing around me.

Initially, I opted for the easy route and obtained a prescription from my female GP. Several years later, experts changed their minds and announced that estrogen no longer protected me from heart attacks, breast cancer and accordion players. "Is it hot in here or is it me?" became my day's lyrics once again, and I bought a huge bottle of the foul-tasting herbal elixir Menopeace, lovingly crafted by my son. He had a few more dollars in his pocket, and my hot flashes disappeared.

But the accordion players haven't. That's because I moved from Oregon to Sweden, and therein lies the real cure for my "change of life."

Because I took the term seriously. After a twenty-year separation during which we'd lost track of one another, the Internet reunited me with my long-lost Swedish sweetheart. We were both available, though reconciled to living alone the rest of our lives. Relationships, we'd decided, just didn't work out for us.

Until we found each other again. Suddenly, late

middle age disappeared and we were teenagers once more, reinventing sex and the flush of fresh love. I moved and we married. I'm still often flushed, but for better reasons. Sure, my skin is dry and I'm finding out why mature women often wear neck scarves. And I'm forgetting just who I went to that prom with. But hey, life's still an adventure, and now I appreciate it more.

Is it happy in here, or is it just me?

♥ *Jann Mitchell*

Spice Up Your Sex Life

With all the physical and emotional changes during menopause, it's not surprising that your sex life may change, too. But it's certainly not true that menopause means the end of a satisfying sex life. You should expect—and you deserve—an active, enjoyable sex life for many years to come.

Yes, you might find that you are less interested in having sex during and after menopause—either because you find it's painful or because you're feeling stressed. Or maybe after many years with the same partner, your lovemaking has gone from exciting to routine. If you have these problems, remember that you can deal with them.

On the other hand, you may be one of the many women who finds your sex life has improved because you no longer have to worry about pregnancy or being interrupted by children at home. And if your partner is slowing down, that can be a good thing—more time for enjoyment!

It's important to remember that even if you're skipping periods, pregnancy is still possible during perimenopause—so unless you're trying to have a baby, be sure to use birth control until you've had no periods for twelve months or when your doctor tells you it's okay.

Sex-related problems can be due to a number of things, including

- **Physical changes.** Decreasing hormone levels can cause body changes that lead to vaginal dryness or pain during sex.
- **Illnesses.** Heart problems, high blood pressure, arthritis, bladder problems or depression all can lead to decreased sexual desire.
- **Drugs.** Many medications can affect sexual function, including some for high blood pressure, antidepressants, sleeping pills and tranquilizers.
- **Menopause symptoms.** Hot flashes, poor sleep and anxiety can get in the way of your ability to enjoy sex.
- **Cultural issues.** There are many conflicting cultural messages about sexuality. These messages influence how a woman views her sexual self, including her body image, role, power and her view of her partner.

Dealing with Physical Changes

- **Treat vaginal dryness.** Try over-the-counter vaginal lubricants.
- **Stay sexually active.** Having sex at least once a week keeps vaginal tissue healthy.
- **Ask your doctor about prescription estrogen—containing creams or vaginal**

suppositories. They are applied directly to the vagina, so less estrogen gets into your system.

- **Eat a healthy diet and exercise.** If you feel overweight and unattractive, that's bound to have an effect on your sexual desire. Keeping fit will make you feel better and look better— a turn-on for both you and your partner.

Dealing with Emotional Changes

As you get older, your idea of a sexy, romantic encounter is likely to change. That's to be expected, and it's not a reflection on your sexuality. If you can't remember the last time you and your partner had a romantic evening, now's the perfect time to change that. Go ahead, use menopause as an excuse to spice up your life. Show him that menopausal mood changes can be a good thing!

Don't Want Sex? Get Help!

If you find that your sex drive has plummeted, and you and your doctor have ruled out physical reasons, you may want to explore counseling with a licensed counselor or therapist. You shouldn't just assume that a flagging sex drive is normal at menopause and should be accepted as a natural part of growing older—it shouldn't be.

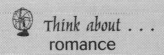
Think about . . .
romance

Instead of worrying about your sexual life, do something about it. Check off these items as you do them—and try to do them all the next couple of months!

❑ Rent a sexy movie.

❑ Get a book on improving your sex life.

❑ Take a shower or bath with your partner.

❑ Buy some sexy lingerie.

❑ Buy candles and some sexy music for the bedroom.

❑ Give your partner a sensual massage and ask for one in return.

❑ Take a warm bath to help you relax.

❑ Take a vacation—you'll unwind and have more time for each other!

My personal favorite ways of enhancing my sex life:

❑ _____

❑ _____

❑ _____

THIS Is a Hot Flash

Sitting with Mary at her church's women's circle meeting one morning, I smiled when one of her friends kidded her about opening the nearby door for a breeze during her hot flashes. It made me think of my mother.

I missed my mother, who in her later years had swiftly lost ground in battling early onset senility. Attending church groups was something she had enjoyed heartily, baking fresh muffins and brewing coffee for every meeting. I had hoped she would be able to enjoy her high-spirited, loving grandchildren and looked forward to attending meetings with her, but it was not to be. Instead, I drove her to countless doctors' offices and helped evaluate nursing homes when she became too frail for my father to manage alone.

I enjoyed the cool breeze from the door. It smelled like the spring day when my mother announced in a trembling voice that she was having a hot flash. She smiled, took my hand in hers and said, "This is a hot flash. It doesn't hurt, but it's a surprise." Her hand felt warm and dry in my own. At twenty-something, I was a determined and ambitious graduate student living at home again, chafing at my chosen poverty status but not at being home again with my parents. "Here comes another one. Mine come in waves. Not everyone's do. Muriel is up at night. Sometimes she has to change her sheets. Grace hardly ever gets them." She sighed, sat back down with her tea. "So, you wear cotton. You dress in layers. You sit near the window. Now, what were you just saying about that professor who's trying to date the girls?"

My mother suffered through graduate school with me. She encouraged me during final exams and when I struggled through finance class. She and my father had an easy familiarity with each other and frank affection I had never seen as a child or a teenager living under their roof. When I had a tumultuous breakup of yet another romance, my mother brewed tea and told me that maybe the ugly ones at school were going to strike it rich and maybe they would be great lovers.

Around this time, my mother let her hair go soft and gray from its rigid black waves. She laughed more often and sang under her breath while she washed the dishes. Sometimes she would ask for help in finishing the crossword puzzles that she worked on at night when she couldn't sleep. Now and again with her hands trembling slightly, she would smile at me and say, "It's another one of those hot flashes!"

One night, when I was forty-four, I woke in the middle of the night feeling very warm and damp in the cotton sheets. My husband snored beside me undisturbed. The house was dark and quiet. Gradually I fell back to sleep, but not before several more waves of this unfamiliar and strange warmth swept over me.

After several nights, I finally realized what was happening. These were hot flashes. They didn't hurt. They sure were a surprise. Within a week, they had subsided. Every now and then I go through a week with several episodes. I know to wear cotton in layers and to sit near the windows. Because I had my children late in life and my daughter is still very young, I won't have the chance to grab her hand and say "This is a hot flash" when it happens. But I will make sure that I tell her about the windows and wearing cotton layers.

♥ *Louise Foerster*

Hormone Therapy

Until fairly recently, most women going through menopause were routinely advised to take hormone therapy to treat symptoms like hot flashes and to protect their bones, heart and memory. Women who had not had a hysterectomy had been given estrogen plus progestin, which is a hormone that protects against cancer of the uterus. Women who had had a hysterectomy had been given estrogen alone.

Then in July 2002, a study of 16,000 women called the Women's Health Initiative (WHI) was halted three years early when preliminary results showed that hormone therapy consisting of a combination of estrogen plus progestin slightly increased women's risk of breast cancer, heart disease, blood clots and stroke. Hormone therapy also has been shown to increase the risk of dementia.

The problem, of course, is that no one knows ahead of time which women will suffer dangerous consequences. That's why many doctors have stopped prescribing hormone therapy for all women just to be safe.

While the risks of hormone therapy are small, they are very real. Having a heart attack or stroke isn't like getting an upset stomach or headache—these are life-altering, potentially disabling events.

So while the decision is ultimately up to the patient, you need to know the risks.

The U.S. Food and Drug Administration now recommends that if you choose to use hormones to relieve your menopause symptoms, you should:

- Only do so if your symptoms are severe
- Take the lowest dose and for the shortest possible time
- Have yearly breast exams by a health care provider, perform monthly breast self-exams and receive periodic mammograms

Hormones for Hot Flashes?

A major reason why women want to take hormone therapy is to stop hot flashes. If you are considering this, ask yourself:

- How frequent and intense are the hot flashes?
- Do they occur at night?
- Have I tried anything else to stop them? How have those solutions worked?
- Do I understand the risks of taking hormone therapy?

If you are having moderate to severe hot flashes that are interfering with your life, and you can't find any effective alternatives, consider using hormones at the lowest possible dose. If you decide to take hormones, every three to six months reassess to see if you're through the worst of the hot flashes. If so, slowly lower the dose over one to two years so there's no shock to the system. In general, by the time a woman is fifty-four or fifty-five, she should be off the hormones.

As with any treatment, you need to carefully weigh your personal risks against the possible benefits and make your choice according to your own health and lifestyle needs. Remember, the decision to take hormones or not is yours—if you feel your doctor isn't listening to your needs and concerns, feel free to talk to another doctor.

Think about . . .
hormone therapy

It can be difficult to decide whether you want to take hormone therapy during menopause. Ask your doctor these questions about hormone therapy:

Why should I take hormone therapy?

What are my risks for heart disease, breast cancer and osteoporosis?

Is there an alternative therapy that I can use short- or long-term?

What alternatives can help me prevent heart disease?

What alternatives can help me prevent osteoporosis?

Have I tried all the other options?

Are the risks—however slight—worth the rewards?

My Page

My Thoughts _____

_____

_____

_____

My Feelings _____

_____

_____

_____

My Facts _____

_____

_____

_____

My Support _____

_____

_____

_____

I'm Flush with Life

I felt myself flushing all of a sudden. I was breaking out in sweat just standing there at the fruit vendor's stall. I looked at him quickly. Well, he was quite good-looking in a rustic way. He did have a gentle, caring look about him, quite unlike the brash, in-your-face approach of today's youth. "Today's youth," that very phrase aged me. I was not experiencing my first flush of excitement at the sight of an attractive member of the opposite sex as an eighteen-year-old might have done. What I was undergoing was definitely hormonal, but at age forty-eight, this flushing was the work of a very different category of hormones than the ones that cause sexual excitement.

This sweating and flushing could also not be attributed to summer heat, since the day was quite chilly, with a strong wind sweeping everything off its feet except women such as me. I stood my ground and sweated it out in the face of the cold wind. Part of my flushing could be due to embarrassment; I still wasn't used to the erratic behavior of my internal thermostat.

My walk had changed from the smooth, gliding one of a twenty-five-year-old to a rather wobbly variety, more like that of a waddling duck. I was often a sitting duck as well, meaning once I sat, very little could move me from my perch. Getting up required a lot of effort, as did sitting down. Moreover, there were always other sweet young things like nieces and nephews to run errands for me while I sat in the sun and enjoyed my cup of tea, the winter sun warming my back and making me forget the nagging aches and pains that my calcium-depleted bones subjected me to. No longer did I have to run around like a sprightly maid, and I was happy to sit and give orders for a change.

Unfortunately, though I feel I have developed a thick skin with time and experience, I flare up unaccountably at times. Blood pressure, my dear! That is why I have wisely joined a yoga group. Here, I've made many friends. As the word "OM" resonates off the walls of the room where our class is held, I feel quite relaxed. The lotus posture is meant for the younger flowers present in the class, but even the older ones do manage to stretch a bit and feel more alive after the class is over. I carry the "OM" word home, and repeat it oft when I feel I need to cool off. "O-O-O-M, SHA-A-A-NTI, O-O-O-M" I go, and the house fills with this chant. The first time I did this, my bewildered dog hid under the bed. Now he just wags his tail. He sits quietly by my side as I go through the various yoga postures. I stretch and unwind as I go through the paces, and I finally do the "Shavasana" (which means to be as still and resting as a corpse). I feel the waves of peace wash over me. It is a period of eternal calm.

Once a week I call my friends over for a game of cards and coffee. My husband happily goes for an evening out with his friends. My friends discuss with me the finer points of anti-aging creams, their battle with bulges, and their desire for sweet-somethings to eat now that the days of whispered sweet-nothings are over for several of them. We laugh as we reminisce of our days gone by, when we thought chocolates and sweet valentines would be there forever. There is a touch of sadness in our talk, because who doesn't miss the brash delight of youth? I remember strutting around as a heady teen, and it somehow doesn't seem that long ago. At the same time, we see young mothers struggling with diapers and milk bottles and thank our lucky stars that those sleepless nights with babies are over. We can sit perched with our coffees and books and read late into the night till our eyes start watering with the strain. We don't have to rush off home to attend to the demands of young children.

Yes, I can now sit and work on the computer, do

my yoga, go for walks and meet with friends, things that I couldn't do when the children were young and demanding. I don't smoke and am not diabetic, so I can afford an occasional lemon tart, even though it goes straight to my waist. I cannot jump and skip but I can enjoy a walk in the park like anyone else. If I don't get amorous glances, I do get greetings of respect which I acknowledge with grace. I can give advice and know it is heeded as the voice of experience. If I have gained in years and weight, I have lost my impatience, my boorishness, my drive towards things to be absolutely "so." I am more relaxed, and the stray gray hairs add sophistication to my look. I have time for myself. I have retained my sense of humor and my sense of self. If my children are now busy with their lives, so am I. I am an independent individual, and cherish the time spent with myself, and with my husband.

My hot flush has subsided, and the nice gentleman who helps me across the street gives me a look of appreciation so sweet that it makes my day. I smile back at him, my eyes twinkling with pleasure. Maybe I can still knock them over, if not off their feet.

♥ *Abha Iyengar*

Alternatives to Hormone Therapy

Given the risks and uncertainties of hormone therapy, you may be looking for non-hormone alternatives to ease your hot flashes and other menopause symptoms. There are quite a few to choose from—from lifestyle changes to dietary supplements. It's important to note that dietary products that can be bought without a prescription are not regulated by the U.S. Food and Drug Administration and therefore their safety and effectiveness have not been evaluated by scientific methods. Be sure to consult your doctor before taking any herbal treatments or dietary supplements—herbal products can interfere or interact with other medications you may be taking.

Non-Hormone Alternatives

Antidepressants

Several major studies have shown that drugs such as Effexor, Paxil and Prozac have been shown to be moderately effective in relieving hot flashes, but the U.S. Food and Drug Administration has not approved antidepressants for this specific use.

Black cohosh

Black cohosh—originally an American Indian remedy—has shown some promise in relieving hot flashes, but it is generally not recommended for use longer than six months.

Soy

Studies have shown that Japanese women, who consume a lot of soy products, are much less likely than women in Western countries to have hot flashes. Soy contains phytoestrogens, which are estrogen-like substances derived from beans, particularly soybeans. Soy seems to be moderately helpful in relieving hot flashes, but studies have not been conclusive. Phytoestrogens from soy can be consumed through foods or supplements. Soy food products include tofu, tempeh, soy milk, and soy nuts and are presumed safe when consumed in this form. There can be no presumption of safety for soy supplements.

Alternative treatments to avoid

Dietary supplements that have not been found effective include dong quai, red clover, wild and Mexican yam, evening primrose oil, vitamin E and acupuncture.

Take Care of Your Health

Your body is going through a lot of changes during menopause. At the same time, you are also getting to the age when your body can become more vulnerable to a number of diseases, like heart disease, osteoporosis, breast cancer and Alzheimer's. But it doesn't have to be that way. Use this time of changes to make positive changes to improve your health—it's the perfect time!

The advice isn't complex, but it's also not easy: quit smoking, eat healthy, reduce stress and get regular exercise.

Heart Disease

While younger women have a lower risk of heart disease than men of the same age, once women hit menopause, their risk is almost the same as men's, so:

- **Get your blood pressure and cholesterol monitored regularly.** High blood pressure increases the risk of heart disease and stroke. It is especially dangerous because often it doesn't have any warning signs or symptoms. Anyone, no matter what their race, age, or gender, can develop high blood pressure. And once you develop high blood pressure, you usually have it for life.

- **Get tested for diabetes.** If you haven't been tested for diabetes, it's time now—and if you do have diabetes, it's important to follow your doctor's treatment plan closely. But the most common type of diabetes, type 2 diabetes, often can be controlled—or even cured.

Osteoporosis

Another common consequence of aging for women is the loss of bone tissue that can weaken your bones and cause osteoporosis. If too much bone is lost, bones become thin and weak and can break easily. The good news is that you can lower your risk of bone loss and osteoporosis if you:

- **Get plenty of calcium and vitamin D.**
- **Do regular weight-bearing exercises like walking, running or dancing.**
- **Ask your doctor if you should be taking medication to prevent bone loss.** Medications are available both to prevent and treat bone loss due to osteoporosis.
- **Protect yourself from falls.** When a woman's bones are weakened by osteoporosis, a fall can cause a break or fracture. Some things you can do to prevent falls include:

  - Use your glasses.

- Ask your doctor if any of the drugs you are taking can make you dizzy or unsteady on your feet.
- Wear rubber-soled and low-heeled shoes.
- Make sure all the rugs and carpeting in your house are firmly attached to the floor, or remove them.
- Use adequate lighting in your home and make sure the floors are clutter-free.
- Use nightlights.

Breast Cancer

There are some positive changes you can make to reduce your risk of breast cancer, such as:

- Cut down on alcohol
- Watch your weight
- Have regular mammograms and manual breast exams.

Women should report any changes in their breasts to their doctor right away. Remember, most of the time, breast changes are not cancer—but only a doctor can tell for sure.

🐝 Think about . . .
my health tests

A thorough physical exam includes a head-to-toe assessment of your health, including the following tests. Ask your doctor how often you need these tests, depending on your age and medical history.

🐝 **Heart Health.** Blood pressure and cholesterol tests—high blood pressure and high cholesterol levels increase your risk of heart disease.

🐝 **Bone Health.** A bone mineral density test is a specialized X-ray scan that measures bone density and fracture risk for osteoporosis.

🐝 **Breast Health.** Your health care provider should do an annual manual examination. You also should receive a mammogram, a low-dose X-ray of the breasts to check for abnormalities (how often you should get one depends on your age and family history of breast cancer).

🐝 **Colon Health.** There are several types of tests, including a blood test and colonoscopy, a test involving a thin, flexible tube that allows the doctor to look into the colon itself.

Reproductive Health. A Pap test tests for pre-cancerous cells or cancer of the cervix or vagina. A pelvic exam is a manual exam of the ovaries and uterus. This is important whether or not you have had a hysterectomy.

Thyroid Health. The thyroid is a gland that controls key functions of your body. Disease of the thyroid gland can affect nearly every organ in your body and harm your health. A thyroid test is a blood test of thyroid hormone levels.

Vision and Hearing Test.

My Page

My Thoughts _____

_____

_____

_____

My Feelings _____

_____

_____

_____

My Facts _____

_____

_____

_____

My Support _____

_____

_____

_____

Hooray—No More "Monthlies"!

My grandmother called her menstrual periods "the monthlies." My mother did, too. So how have I always referred to my special time of the month? Same way, of course.

As in "Can't go swimming—I have my monthly." Or "Can't go camping—I have my monthly." Or "Can't wear that new pair of white shorts that shows off my legs to their best advantage—I have my monthly."

And worst of all "Not tonight, dear. As a matter of fact, not for the next five or six nights. I have my monthly."

I got to thinking not long ago (as I was tossing and turning at 2 A.M., unable to sleep and drenched in sweat even though it was the middle of January) about just how many monthlies I've had in my life. *Let's see,* I said to myself. *I started having periods when I was almost thirteen. I'm closing in on fifty. That's thirty-seven years of monthlies.*

Thirty-seven years? Yikes! Did I dare multiply thirty-seven by twelve months in a year? Sure, I dared. I just couldn't do it in my head. Since I needed to get up anyway to put on a dry night-gown, I grabbed a pencil and scratch pad from the bedside table and went to figuring.

Thirty-seven times twelve equals 444 monthlies. Yikes again! To be fair, I needed to subtract the three times I was pregnant and nursing. I knocked off twelve monthlies for each of those. Then I took away another handful for the rare occasions when I was irregular. That still left almost four hundred weeks out of my life when monthlies put a cramp in my style, so to speak.

Double, triple, quadruple yikes!

I crawled back into bed, head spinning. Having spent the past several months experiencing—and complaining about—hot flashes and night sweats and weight gain and mood swings and all the other negatives that accompany menopause, I had never really paused to consider the upside.

Sure, I was something of a hormonal wreck. But I had been a hormonal wreck once a month *four hundred times.* Maybe it was time to put all that bad-mood experience to work and find ways to adjust my attitude.

And what of all the money I was no longer flushing away? Tampons, pads and ache-pain-bloating medicine set me back at least ten dollars a month. Over the past thirty-seven years, I had probably spent close to four thousand dollars on monthlies. Four thousand dollars! Maybe it was time to start holding back ten dollars each month and buying something totally fun and frivolous—lunch with a friend or a new lipstick or a Sunday matinee with jumbo popcorn-and-drink.

Then there was the lingerie issue. For as long as I could remember, my top dresser drawer had been divided into two sections. One was for "under-pants"—cheap, stained, and ugly garments I wore during my monthlies. The other section was for "panties"—lacy, feminine and oh-so-sexy little numbers that I wore the rest of the time. Into tomorrow's trash the yucky stuff would go, along with the drawer divider.

Sleep was about to claim me. But not before images of all the adventures I'd ever had to turn down rolled through my mind.

The cattle drive out west—cancelled because of my monthly. The long ski weekend in Vermont—cancelled because of my monthly. Ditto to a scuba adventure, a trip in a hot air balloon, and a week hiking the Appalachian Trail.

I pulled the blanket up under my chin and snuggled close to my husband. Yes, this menopause thing was going to require some adjustments. For me, for him, for our three nearly-grown children. But maybe the changes weren't going to be so bad after all.

♥ *Jennie Ivey*

Take Charge of Your Health Care

Menopause is a time of many changes, and many important decisions. While it is ultimately up to you whether you will want hormone therapy, having a strong relationship with your doctor will help you make the best choice for you. Your doctor can help you figure out how to deal with your symptoms and how to work with you to help protect you from the many age-related conditions that you may face in the coming years.

Make a list of your questions before you visit the doctor and refer to the list during your visit. If your doctor says anything you don't understand, ask to have it repeated. If doctor visits tend to overwhelm you, bring along a friend or relative who can take notes, offer support and help ask questions.

Tell your doctor about:

Any herbs or dietary supplements you're taking. Just because you can buy them without a prescription doesn't mean they're harmless.

Your symptoms. Describe your symptoms: when they started, how they make you feel, what triggers them, and what you've done to relieve them.

Your daily habits. Don't be embarrassed—be honest about your diet, physical activity, smoking, alcohol or drug use, and sexual history. Your doctor can't give you the best care if you withhold information.

Ask about:

- **Test results**—how will you find out about them and how long it will take to get them.
- **Side effects** of any medication you've been prescribed. Are there alternatives? How much will it cost, how long will it last and will insurance cover it?
- **How to take the medicine:** what to do if you miss a dose; if there are any foods, drugs or activities you should avoid when taking the medicine; and if there is a generic brand available at a lower price—you can ask your pharmacist these questions, too.

Getting a Second Opinion

There are times when you may not feel comfortable with a particular doctor. Don't dismiss those feelings—you'll need to talk about very intimate and personal things when you're going through menopause, and if you don't feel at ease talking with that person, you may want to consider switching doctors.

Or you may not agree with your doctor's recommendations. In that case, you should think about getting a second opinion. Another doctor might have a different perspective or new options for the treatment of menopause.

Here are some tips on how to get a second opinion:

- Ask your doctor to recommend someone else—either another primary care doctor or a specialist—for another opinion. Don't worry about hurting your doctor's feelings. If you prefer, you can call a hospital or medical society in your area for names of doctors.
- Check with your health insurance provider to see if they cover the cost of a second opinion. Find out if you need a referral from your primary care doctor.
- Have your primary care doctor send medical records to the doctor you're seeing for a second opinion so you don't have to repeat any medical tests. Your primary care doctor's office may charge a fee for this service.
- As with your primary care doctor, come prepared to meet the new doctor with a list of questions and concerns.
- Ask this doctor to send a written report to your primary care doctor, and get a copy for your own records.

Think about . . .
my health

My main health concerns are:

_____

_____

My current status in each of these categories is:

    Heart health _____

    Bone health _____

    Breast health _____

I want to talk to my doctor about:

_____

I'd like a second opinion on:

_____

My worst habits are:

_____

My steps to improve my life are:

_____

_____

Quitting Nic

My affair with nicotine began when I was a sweet-breathed seventeen-year-old. Nic was so cool, and all of the other girls loved him. I wanted Nic, too. From the moment he first touched my lips, he became my ever-present lover. I just couldn't live without him!

Nic seduced me over and over again with promises of serenity and comfort; he made me feel better. He never let me out of his sight and accompanied me everywhere I went. From the moment I woke up to the time I laid my head on my pillow, Nic was by my side. Hand-in-hand we traveled together. Always.

I believed those smoky promises. Over and over again.

Even as he damaged my favorite clothes, left holes in my carpet, burned through hundreds of my hard-earned dollars each month, I forgave him. "It's not a big deal," I'd say. And even when people whose opinions mattered looked at me with a subtle frown, I turned away, agreeing with them. "You're right, it's nasty." But we continued to huddle together in our smoky haze, in the rain, in the cold and in the heat.

Neither my daughter's tears nor my husband's begging could end our relationship. Not doctors telling me our relationship was unhealthy, guaranteeing me he will abandon me to an oxygen tank one day, would loosen the grip. Not even chronic sinusitis with headaches that would put me in bed for a day made me quit.

Yes, Nic and I had our spats. Bullied into leaving him, I'd run back as soon as I could, just waiting for an opportune moment. I was a "hyperquit." Four months here, six weeks there. But Nic preyed on me in my weakest, most sorrowful moments. When my father died and I got the call at 4 A.M., the first thing I did after months away from smoking was go to the store, buy a pack and drive home, smoke and tears clouding my vision.

His voice whispered in my head even when a pack wasn't in my purse. "Just one," he would say. "Just one will make you feel better and then I will leave you alone." Just one visit with Nic, I would think, and then I'll quit. And that one visit turned back into a pack-a-day lifestyle.

Two years ago, I took my husband to the emergency room. His chest was hurting so bad he could barely breathe. He looked at me with pain-filled eyes and said, "No more cigarettes." His pain was caused by acid reflux. And cigarette smoke exacerbated the problem. I was causing my husband to hurt.

Yet I didn't quit immediately. I just moved the habit away from him, guiltily, sadly. I would sit on the porch alone with my cigarettes in a self-imposed exile, thinking. I began to hear new whispers in my head, and they weren't from Nic.

"I hate cigarettes," my husband said. "You're not getting any younger," my doctor reminded me. "Wrinkles are caused by smoke," news stories reported. "Homes that smell of smoke don't sell as well," my Realtor stated.

I couldn't fool myself anymore. This relationship I had was unhealthy and unappealing. Finally, all of the negatives added up to one compelling reason to quit: I wanted to.

And so it happened, after quitting time and again, after so many years of my life devoted to this insidious relationship in my head, I finally stopped. My birthday present to myself was a Nic-free world. Armed with patches, gobs of gum and a steely resolve, I left my hourly visits with a twenty-year companion.

Ending my relationship with nicotine wasn't easy. It was one of the hardest things I've ever done. I felt like I had lost something dear to me, and I even grieved. Like an alcoholic, I know I can never have just one.

But what I've gained is so much more precious. The small things in life that I didn't realize I had missed were huge. Clean air, the smell of freshly laundered sheets. Sweet breath again, whiter teeth. Fast seating in restaurants, the delightful tastes of three different chocolates in my favorite cake, virtually no sinus pain. And my family's pride and respect.

Most of all I have my freedom. I am finally free to live a healthy life. Good-bye, Nic. Yes, I really can live without you.

♥ *Mesa Foard*

Quit Smoking

There are so many reasons for women going through menopause to quit smoking. Not only does smoking increase menopausal symptoms such as hot flashes and urinary incontinence, it also increases the risk of heart disease, lung cancer, emphysema and osteoporosis—not to mention wrinkles!

If you quit smoking you will also:

- Get rid of that annoying morning cough.
- Have more energy.
- Be free of smoky-smelling hair, clothes, car and home.
- Reduce your child's colds, earaches and coughs by removing secondhand smoke from your home.
- Have more control over your life.
- Save money!

My top reasons for quitting are:

_____

_____

_____

Sure, it's hard to quit. Nicotine is a powerful and addictive drug. You've probably tried to quit before, but now that you're committed to making other healthy changes—eating right and exercising—it's a perfect time to give up smoking for good.

How to Quit

- **Pick a quit date.** Before that day, get rid of all your cigarettes, ashtrays and lighters, anywhere you might stash them—don't forget your car!
  My quit date is _____

- **Write down why you want to quit** and keep it in a place where you'll see it.
  I want to quit because_____

  _____

- **When you get the urge to smoke, do something else.** Go for a walk, go to the movies, or call a friend. Exercise, take a bath, or read.
  When I want to smoke I will_____

- **Change your routine.** If you're used to drinking coffee with your cigarette, switch to tea instead. If you usually smoke on your way to work, take a different route.
  I will change my routine by_____

- **Try medication.** Nicotine gums and patches are available over the counter. You also can talk to your doctor about prescription medication to help you quit.
  I'll ask my doctor about _____

- **Look for help.** Your local hospital, wellness center, health department or American Lung Association (*www.lungusa.org*, or 1-800-LUNG-USA) all have resources to help you quit smoking.
  I'll look for help through_____

  _____

- **Reward yourself.** For every week that you don't smoke, do something nice for yourself.
  My reward for not smoking for a week will be

  _____

Where Are the Oreos?

"Where are the Oreos?" my husband asks, his head deep in the pantry.

"Not there," I answer.

"The Ring Dings? The M&Ms? Where is anything to eat that isn't good for you?"

As I grope my way through change-of-life issues, he's learning to cope with change-of-pantry issues. The cans of condensed soup, packages of cookies and boxes of macaroni and cheese have been replaced by legions of vitamins and herbs and shelves of tea. Sugared cereals have given way to granola, candy bars to multigrain bread. Everything is calcium-enriched and isoflavone-enhanced.

Part of this change comes from a general societal shift that recognizes the importance of good nutrition. Rings Dings are not suggested in any of the major food groups and the sodium content in most canned soups would give cows at the salt lick pause. Part of it is a search for a more natural way of eating, free of preservatives and trans fats. Still another part comes from the ecological awareness of limiting excess packaging. All great reasons for stocking up on fiber contained in whole grains and minimally processed foods.

But I must be truthful. The main reason is the needs of this new life stage. My body is shifting. Foods I used to eat without a second thought have turned against me. Sugar gives me headaches. Chocolate sets up cravings that wipe out any idea of real food. Unrefined carbs go straight to my waist and after doing their damage disappear in a New York minute, leaving me with a ravenous hunger and a calorie intake more attuned to a sumo wrestler than to a small, midlife female.

My husband grumbles as he burrows behind the containers of soy milk, dried fruit and protein bars, digging further into the pantry looking for something appetizing.

"Have some chips," I suggest.

"We have chips?"

He reaches for the non-aluminum lined bags to discover taro, baked-not-fried corn, sesame-soy and sweet potato chips.

"We don't have chips," he says as he puts the bags back on the shelf. "We don't have anything edible!" he wails.

"Keep looking," I tell him.

He finally comes up with one of the shiny, crackly, jiggly bags of Ghirardelli double chocolate bits I buy especially for him. His face lights up as he tears into it and pops the bits, one by one, into his mouth, savoring each one as it melts on his tongue.

I may be health conscious and I may be menopausal but I am not cruel. Sometimes a man just needs his chocolate the way a woman needs her soy. My pantry knows it. And so do I.

♥ *Ferida Wolff*

Eat Healthfully

Now's your opportunity to prove to yourself— and others—that middle-age weight gain isn't inevitable! Through a healthy diet, you can protect your bones and heart, and look and feel better. In order for you to make lasting changes to your health, you'll need to make a lifelong commitment to healthy eating.

What constitutes a healthy diet for a woman in the menopause years? Here are the essential ingredients:

Limit saturated fat. Eat foods that are high in monounsaturated fats, such as olive oil, canola oil, nuts and seafood.

Load up on fruits and vegetables. Great nutritional choices include green leafy vegetables, sweet potatoes, oranges, tomatoes, blueberries and squash.

Eat less sodium. Sodium (salt) can raise your blood pressure, which in turn can increase your risk of heart disease. Don't just pour on salt when you're cooking or eating—use herbs and spices instead. Check labels of prepackaged foods to see how much sodium they contain.

You need lots of calcium. You need plenty of calcium to maintain healthy bones and protect against osteoporosis. Calcium-rich foods include low-fat milk and cheese, and broccoli. Many foods are fortified with calcium, such as orange juice, cereals and breakfast bars.

You may also need to take a calcium supplement if you can't get as much as you need from food. Calcium supplements are available without a prescription in a wide range of preparations and strengths. Here are some things to consider in choosing and using a supplement:

- The most common types of calcium supplements are calcium carbonate and calcium citrate. Another type, tribasic calcium phosphate, is also available. Many common antacids also contain calcium.
- When choosing among brands, look for labels that state "purified" or have the USP (United States Pharmacopeia) symbol.
- Avoid calcium from unrefined oyster shell, bone meal or dolomite without the USP, because these may have higher lead levels or other toxic metals.
- Calcium is absorbed best by the body when it is taken several times a day in amounts of 500 mg or less. Calcium carbonate is absorbed best when taken with food. Calcium citrate can be taken any time.

- Calcium supplements must dissolve in the body in order for them to be absorbed and protect bones. Chewable and liquid supplements dissolve well because they are broken down before they enter the stomach. To test how well a tablet dissolves, put one in a small amount of warm water for thirty minutes, stirring it occasionally. If it hasn't dissolved within this time, it probably won't dissolve in your stomach.
- To avoid side effects such as gas or constipation, take 500 mg a day for a week, then add more calcium slowly. If you are feeling side effects, drink more fluids and eat more fiber. Or try another form of calcium.
- Ask your doctor or pharmacist whether your calcium supplement might interfere with anything else you're taking, such as antibiotics or iron supplements.

You also need vitamin D, which absorbs the calcium. You can get vitamin D from fortified dairy products, egg yolks, saltwater fish and liver. Some calcium supplements have vitamin D added.

Another great source of vitamin D is sunlight, so don't be afraid to spend a lot of quality time outdoors.

Eat fiber. The recommended amount is 25 to 30 grams of fiber a day, to help prevent heart disease and strokes. Good food sources of fiber include fruits and vegetables, dried beans, oats and barley. Also eat whole grains (such as whole wheat bread instead of white bread) to help prevent colon cancer and keep your digestive system running smoothly.

And since you're boosting your fiber intake, don't forget to drink lots of water, one of the best and easiest ways to keep your body looking and feeling younger.

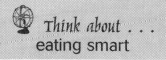

Think about . . .
eating smart

Try three substitutions from this list each week.

Instead of . . .	I will choose . . .
Vegetable oil	Olive or canola oil
Red meat	Seafood or skinless chicken
Hard margarine or butter	Soft unsaturated margarine
Whole milk	Skim milk
Fried foods	Baked, steamed, boiled or broiled
Sour cream and mayonnaise	Plain low-fat yogurt
Sauces, butter and salt	Herbs and spices
Regular hard and processed cheeses	Low-fat, low-sodium cheeses
Salted crackers	Unsalted or low-sodium whole-wheat crackers
Salted potato chips	Unsalted tortilla, unsalted pretzels and popcorn

Dining Out

If your family is like most, you don't have time to prepare home-cooked meals every night. Eating out may well be a regular part of your meal plan. But that's no excuse for not sticking to your new healthy way of eating! With a little creativity and some advance planning, you can almost always find a way to eat a healthy meal while dining out.

- **Avoid the bread basket.** Those rolls are probably made from refined flour that contain no nutrients or fiber. For this reason sandwiches are not a good choice unless you skip the bread.

- **Eat salads, both as appetizers and as your entrée.** If you choose a salad as your main entrée, be sure to add proteins such as chicken, fish and eggs, and fats such as avocado. Ask for your salad dressing on the side and stick to the vinaigrettes instead of creamy dressings.

- 🌀 **Choose foods that are steamed, broiled, baked, roasted, poached or stir-fried.**
- 🌀 **Share food,** such as a main dish or dessert, with your dining partner.
- 🌀 **Take part of the food home with you, and refrigerate immediately.** To make sure you have leftovers, ask for a take-home container when the meal arrives. Put half the meal into it, so you're more likely to eat only what's left on your plate.
- 🌀 **Ask that your meal be served without gravy, sauces, butter or margarine.**
- 🌀 **Remember you don't have to clean your plate**—some restaurants serve enormous portions!

Rites of Passage

"Did you turn up the thermostat?" I asked my husband as I wiped rivulets of perspiration from my face. We sat across from each other at the breakfast table. Clean-shaven and fresh from his shower, he was dressed in his tie, shirt and suit, ready for work. "No." He seemed surprised by my question. "Why did you ask? Are you too hot?" I wiggled out of my robe wondering why he asked such a stupid question. Couldn't he see that I had turned into a waterfall?

He winked and flashed a seductive grin. "Are you trying to make me late for work?" Was he crazy? I could hardly wait for him to finish eating his breakfast and leave so I could rinse off in the shower. "I think I'm having hot flashes," I grumbled. He stopped in mid-bite. "Have you talked to your doctor?" "Not yet, but I've got an appointment later this week," I assured him.

I kept my medical appointment and received confirmation that I had earned membership in the legion of ladies beginning the rite of passage into menopause.

Determined to control the erratic battle between my estrogen and testosterone hormones, I decided to avoid medication. I'd let mind-over-matter be my armament. Up until then I naively believed that men sweated and women perspired. I quickly realized there is no difference. Sweat is sweat and the way water gushed from my pores during hot flashes made me feel like a hot water faucet stuck at the open position.

My husband's mother had died of a heart attack during her menopause so he was extremely concerned about my health. Accustomed to business conferences, he assembled our teenaged daughters around our kitchen table and explained to them that I was experiencing hormonal eruptions. "We must all be careful not to upset your mother. She's going through what's called menopause and must avoid stress. It's an affliction that happens to older women."

I bit down on my lip and withheld comment. He meant well, but his reference to me as an older woman had just defeated years of my zealous efforts to portray a young image to our daughters.

It was a very somber occasion until our youngest asked, with youthful innocence, "If women go through menopause do men go through woman-pause?" We all laughed while he denied it, but it did conclude the discussion.

After that, our girls took great care not to agitate me. Much to my dismay, there were many times when I wished they would, so I had an excuse to vent my emotional frustrations.

Because they didn't, I had no justification to complain about all the extra laundry, much of it caused by my night sweats. Every morning I arose to see my damp silhouette outlined on my sheet. While I did enjoy losing weight from water loss I didn't enjoy feeling like a sponge in my sodden nightgown.

Competing with the hot flashes were the unpredictable bursts of energy that sent me into perpetual motion. Because frequent dreams are another symptom of menopause, I paid diligent attention to mine. I knew that dreaming about houses refers to the dreamer's body, so I interpreted that to mean I should redecorate our house.

My devoted husband gave me carte blanche. So I spent several months painting walls, sewing draperies, and supervising new carpet installation. By completion of that project, my energy level had stabilized enough for me to resume my lifelong enjoyment of reading. That's when I discovered the historical significance of belly dancing, which, prior to then I considered eroticism. Now I realized that this five-thousand-year-old Arabic dance was an art form depicting the difference between good and evil as represented by the snake and swan.

Eager to share this knowledge, I convinced our local recreation department to start a class. I was greatly gratified when over seventy women, eager to ward off evil in our community, enrolled.

Then my husband was promoted and we were transferred to a city back in the Midwest. Our house sold quickly, thanks to my redecorating. By the time we had relocated and settled into our new home my hormones had calmed down. I had survived menopause!

One morning at breakfast in our new kitchen, my husband raised his coffee cup to his lips at the same time I mentioned, "Today I plan to enroll in an advanced belly-dancing class."

His hand shook so radically he spilled his coffee. Always tidy, he reached for his napkin. But instead of mopping up his spilled coffee, he wiped rivulets of sweat from his face. "Did you turn up the thermostat?"

That was the day I learned our daughter was right. Men do go through womanpause.

♥ *Sally Kelly-Engeman*

Get Fit!

A regular program of physical activity can help you manage the symptoms of menopause like hot flashes, decrease your risk of health problems like heart disease and osteoporosis, help you lose weight, and make you feel good—isn't that enough reason to get off the couch?

Exercise also improves your mood and relieves stress—essential during the menopause years. And it can help head off sleep problems, another major bonus.

The best kind of exercise program combines weight-bearing aerobic activity (such as walking), with strength training (weights, resistance bands, yoga or even gardening), and stretching. The key is consistency—try to do some moderate activity every day, or at least most days of the week.

Some Good Exercise Choices

- **Walking** is a great way to get started on exercise, especially if you haven't exercised before or have a lot of weight to lose. At first, don't worry about speed. If you can't talk when you're walking, you're going too fast! Once you're comfortable with your walking routine, try using handheld weights to combine aerobic activity with strength training.

- **Exercise videos** provide privacy, while allowing you to choose the music, instructor and type of exercise. Consider buying handheld weights to combine aerobic and strength exercises.
- **Aerobic dance** is a great way to get fit and meet new people. Many aerobic classes incorporate weights, which is most beneficial for weight loss. **Low-impact aerobics,** in which one foot is always on the ground (no jumping or running in place) is safer.
- **Swimming exercises** your whole body and won't overstress your muscles and joints. Pushing the water away from you provides natural resistance that builds up your muscles. You can add to the resistance effect by using handheld paddles.

Here are some other ideas to get you started:

- Begin and end at a slightly slower pace to warm up and cool down. Do stretching exercises after each session.
- If thirty minutes of exercise all at once seems too overwhelming, split it up into shorter periods—ten minutes, three times a day.
- Choose activities you enjoy and can fit into your daily schedule. Don't choose a morning swim routine if you hate getting up early.

- Don't worry if you miss a day or two—just do your best to make exercise a regular part of your life. Soon you'll realize you don't feel as good if you don't exercise!
- Find someone who will exercise with you.

Choosing a Gym

If you're the type of person who finds it motivating to exercise in a group, then you'll want to look into joining a gym or a local Y. You don't have to spend a lot of money to find a nice, clean place to exercise—many communities have low-cost community centers that offer a gym and workout classes. Don't choose a facility that's too far away—you may be motivated to go now, but will you still want to drive there three times a week next winter? Is the facility's schedule convenient for you? Visit at the time of day you're most likely to go, and see whether there's a long wait for the equipment you want to use. Are there staff members available to show you how to correctly use the equipment?

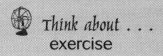

Think about . . .
exercise

My favorite exercises are:

❑ Walking

❑ Jogging

❑ Aerobics

❑ Swimming

❑ Tennis

❑ Bicycle riding

❑ Going to the gym

❑ Belly dancing

❑ Other:

_____

_____

_____

My exercise goal is:

_____minutes a day

_____times a week

The Woman on the Mountain

When I first felt the alchemy of menopause rearranging my body, my mind and my emotions, I wanted to ask questions.

It was the early 1980s. Back then, there were few books or articles about menopause except medical or psychiatric ones. I could find no one to consult. My mother had experienced merely the sudden cessation of her bleeding. Not even one hot flash, let alone episodes of crankiness, forgetfulness or foggy brain, and least of all a deep, inner questioning of her life's purpose or an uprush of grief over some unnamed loss. She had never suffered from PMS either. In her eyes I was, I think, rather odd and strange.

Even the oldest among my friends were younger than me. There was no one to give me advice. So my journey through menopause was a lonely one—at first. Then, help came unexpectedly.

One afternoon, when clouds of depression were swirling around me so thickly that I felt suicidal, I wrapped myself up in a blanket and lay down in the middle of the living-room floor. Outside, the sun was shining. But I was deep in a world of inner turmoil, storm and tumult, incoherent thought, and fearsome blackness. I closed my eyes and drew myself into a tight ball, feeling utterly forsaken and alone, lost in a night forest.

Drifting in my personal darkness, with this image of being lost in a forest, I suddenly saw, with my inner eyes, a flight of worn, stone steps leading upwards through the undergrowth. I began to climb.

Dragging myself up, limbs heavy with weariness, passing through ferns that brushed my face and body, I eventually came out onto a rocky ledge. I seemed to be quite high up, on a mountain. Immediately ahead of me was a large, granite out-crop with clear sky behind it. And standing quietly, motionless in the shadow of the massive rocks, was the figure of a woman.

I had no idea who she was. I could not even see her clearly. But I found myself running desperately towards her, crying.

The next moment, I was in her arms. As she held me, soothed me, stroked my hair, my whole being became suffused with her love. It was the most complete and healing embrace I had ever known. My mother may perhaps have held me like that once, back in my early babyhood, before I grew into the boisterous, scampering child who caused her innate, British reserve to reassert itself. But I could not consciously remember having felt as loved and cherished in my entire life as I did in this strange woman's arms.

As she held me, I felt the surprising slimness and lightness of her body. She was as light as an autumn leaf, with brown skin, smooth and worn, dry, yet soft like an old leather glove, and smelling faintly of patchouli.

The fabric of her dress was identical to the favorite Indian caftan I had worn around the house back in the late 1960s, when I was at my peak of vibrant, strong, confident womanhood, mothering my young daughters, happy and glowing. But she was an old woman. Old, and very, very wise.

She spoke to me softly, soothing me, reassuring me with her words. She whispered her name to me. A name she said I must never divulge. It was a strange, Mexican-sounding name. I must commit this name to memory, she said. In the future, any time I needed her comfort or counsel, all I had to do was call her name and search for the stone steps, and she would always be waiting there, at the top, by the rocks.

And she was.

I went often to that place, after that day, and always she would be there, just as she had promised. Always, she held me in her slim arms and whispered words of wise counsel in my ear. And every time, I came back refreshed, renewed, encouraged, and feeling deeply loved and supported.

One day, she took me to the edge of the mountain ledge and showed me another path. This one led down across a gently sloping, grassy meadow into a beautiful valley. In the valley was a little town with a church spire. It looked so peaceful. I felt a strong yearning to go there, to walk down that meadow path in the sunshine. But she told me it was not yet time.

All this while, in the outer world, I was back at graduate school. I had chosen for my research topic that which I most desperately wanted to understand—the psychological and spiritual aspects of menopause. So while my busy mind was studying the dynamics of this highly significant phase in my life and in the lives of all the other scores of women I was interviewing, my body and my spirit were living its days, struggling through its sweaty nights, and learning all it had to teach. Moments of clarity were interspersed with times of menopausal fog, inexplicable tears and strange aches and pains, sending me scurrying back to the mountain. My college supervisors had no idea that they shared their supervisory task with a mysterious old woman whose face they had never seen. In fact, I had never seen it either. She was not a face to me but a feeling, a texture, a scent, a sense of rightness, an all-enfolding, healing love. Her guidance was invaluable. Without it, I would have felt totally lost.

The months lengthened into years. My thesis was eventually completed and I was determined that the material it was made of would one day be rewoven into a book for other women to read. The hot flashes grew less and less frequent and finally ceased altogether. My body grew lighter, softer, more peaceful to be in. My mind became calm. Energy returned. New possibilities began to arise. I felt like a phoenix, newly arisen from what was now a pile of cooling ash.

One day, I realized with a shock that it had been many, many months since I had visited the woman on the mountain. I felt guilty, as though I had deserted her.

I hurried up the steps, almost expecting to find the place empty. But she was still there, standing quietly as always. We embraced.

This time, however, instead of holding me and whispering, she took my hands silently in hers and held me at arm's length, smiling. As I saw her face for the first time, I got the shock of my life.

It was identical to mine.

A second later, I found myself alone on the mountain. Alone, but not in the least lonely, nor afraid.

I hesitated for a brief moment and then began to walk down the path through the meadow, singing, swinging my arms in the sunshine as I moved toward the little town and out into my new life.

♥ *Marian Van Eyk McCain*

You're on Your Way

So now you're as prepared as you can be. You know the range of symptoms you may encounter and have lots of ideas for how to handle them. You've given serious thought to how to talk to friends and family about menopause, and you're ready to tackle stress head-on. Not content to let things in the bedroom slide, you're willing to take risks and try new things to spice up your sex life.

While you may not have decided yet about whether to take hormones for your menopause symptoms, you know what the issues are and how to talk about it with your doctor. You're eager to start making changes to improve your health, including eating healthfully and exercising regularly.

So what's next? Living life to the fullest! Take this opportunity to jot down some things you've always wanted to do.

Here's a hobby I'd like to try:

_____

_____

Here's a class I'd like to take:

_____

_____

Here's a trip I'd like to make:

_____

_____

Here's a friend I haven't seen in a long time whom I'm going to make a date with:

_____

_____

Here's something I'd like to do with my husband:

_____

_____

Okay, now you have it in writing . . . it's up to you to make it happen. Enjoy!

Resources

The American College of Obstetricians and Gynecologists (ACOG) publishes a number of pamphlets about menopause and related topics. Contact them at:

409 12th Street, SW
Box 96920
Washington, DC 20090
Phone: 202-638-5577
Web site: *www.acog.org*

National Cancer Institute (NCI)
Cancer Information Service (CIS) provides fact sheets and publications about many types of cancer of concern to women in their menopausal years. Contact them at:

Phone: 1-800-4-CANCER (1-800-422-6237)
TTY: 1-800-332-8615
Web site: *http://cis.nci.nih.gov*

The National Heart, Lung, and Blood Institute (NHLBI) Information Center provides information on postmenopausal hormone therapy. Contact them at:

Box 30105
Bethesda, MD 20824
Phone: 301-592-8573
TTY: 240-629-3255
Web site: *www.nhlbi.nih.gov*

The National Institute on Aging (NIA) offers free information on health and aging. For a complete list of publications contact:

NIA Information Center
PO Box 8057
Gaithersburg, MD 20898-8057

Phone: 1-800-222-2225
TTY: 1-800-222-4225
Web site: *www.nia.nih.gov*

NIH Osteoporosis and Related Bone Diseases—National Resource Center provides information on osteoporosis, including fact sheets in Spanish and Asian languages. Contact them at:

1232 22nd Street, NW
Washington, DC 20037-1292
Phone: 1-800-624-BONE
(1-800-624-3663)
Web site: *www.osteo.org*

National Osteoporosis Foundation provides information on preventing and treating osteoporosis. Contact them at:

1232 22nd Street, NW
Washington, DC 20037-1292
Phone: 202-223-2226
Web site: *http://www.nof.org*

National Women's Health Resource Center encourages women to embrace healthy lifestyles to promote wellness and prevent disease. Their website provides information on menopause and related health conditions. Contact them at:

157 Broad Street, Suite 315
Red Bank, NJ 07701
Phone: 1-877-986-9472
Web site: *http://www.healthywomen.org*

North American Menopause Society website contains information on perimenopause, early menopause, menopause symptoms and long-term health effects of estrogen loss, and a wide variety of therapies to enhance health. Contact them at:

Box 94527
Cleveland, OH 44101
Phone: 440-442-7550
Web site: *www.menopause.org*

Planned Parenthood Federation of America, Inc. offers information on menopause including a document on their website titled "Menopause—Another Change in Life." Contact them at:

810 Seventh Avenue
New York, NY 10019
Phone: 1-800-230-PLAN (1-800-230-7526)
Web site: *www.plannedparenthood.org*

Women's Health Initiative (WHI) is a major fifteen-year research program to address the most common causes of death, disability and poor quality of life in post-menopausal women—cardiovascular disease, cancer, and osteoporosis. Results of the WHI Postmenopausal Hormone Therapy Trials are available on their website. Contact them at:

1 Rockledge Centre, Suite 300
MSC 7966
6705 Rockledge Drive
Bethesda, MD 20892-7966
Phone: 301-402-2900
Web site: *www.nhlbi.nih.gov/whi*

Who is Jack Canfield,
Co-Creator of *Chicken Soup for the Soul*?

Jack Canfield is one of America's leading experts in the development of human potential and personal effectiveness. He is both a dynamic, entertaining speaker and a highly sought-after trainer. Jack has a wonderful ability to inform and inspire audiences toward increased levels of self-esteem and peak performance. He has authored or co-authored numerous books, including *Dare to Win, The Aladdin Factor, 100 Ways to Build Self-Concept in the Classroom, Heart at Work* and *The Power of Focus.* His latest book is *The Success Principles.*

www.jackcanfield.com

Who is Mark Victor Hansen,
Co-Creator of *Chicken Soup for the Soul*?

In the area of human potential, no one is more respected than Mark Victor Hansen. For more than thirty years, Mark has focused solely on helping people from all walks of life reshape their personal vision of what's possible. His powerful messages of possibility, opportunity and action have created powerful change in thousands of organizations and millions of individuals worldwide. He is a prolific writer of bestselling books such as *The One Minute Millionaire, The Power of Focus, The Aladdin Factor* and *Dare to Win.*

www.markvictorhansen.com

Who is Susan L. Hendrix, D.O.?

Susan L. Hendrix, D.O., is Professor of Obstetrics and Gynecology at the Wayne State University School of Medicine in Detroit, Michigan. She is Director and Principal Investigator of the National Institutes of Health-sponsored Women's Health Initiative at Wayne State University. Her primary focus is on the causes, prevention and treatment of major diseases affecting women, including heart disease, cancer and osteoporosis. She has a large clinical practice in menopause. Dr. Hendrix has received many awards including being the only physician recognized by the Michigan Women's Commission and Governor John Engler as an honoree of "30 Years, 30 Women."

Who is Celia Slom Vimont (writer)?

Celia Slom Vimont is a health and medical writer. A graduate of the Columbia School of Journalism, she has written for magazines, newspapers and wire services for both consumers and physicians. The former Director of Editorial Services for the American Lung Association, Celia served as in-house editor for books on asthma and smoking cessation for the association and continues to write about a variety of lung health issues. Celia lives in New York City with her husband and son.

Contributors

Criss Bertling is a freelance writer and women's event speaker in South Florida as well as Director of Communications and Women's Ministry at Spanish River Church in Boca Raton, FL. Her website is *www.crissbertling.com.*

Marcia Byalick is a young adult novelist and columnist for a Long Island, N.Y. magazine called *Distinction.* She loves working both as the content editor of *www.beinggirl.com,* a website for teenage girls, and a teacher of memoir writing for adults who want to get the story of their lives down on paper.

Jenna Cassell is a freelance writer, independent consultant, media producer, educator, interpreter, and founder of an American Sign Language media company. She has received over twenty media production awards and is included in multiple *Who's Who.* Jenna can be reached by e-mail: *jencass@san.rr.com.*

Deborah Bates Cavitt went through menopause at age 31, twenty years ago. Deborah has been a school librarian for over twenty-five years. She has written several public relations articles, book reviews, and lesson plans for Linworth Publishing. She is a reviewer for Christian Library Journal. She has published a poem about her Grandpa Ealey in *Weeones* e-zine and has a selection in *Chicken Soup for the Grandmother's Soul.*

Harriet Cooper is a freelance humorist and essayist living in Toronto, Canada. Her humor, essays, articles, short stories and poetry have appeared in national and international newspapers, magazines, Web sites, newsletters, anthologies, radio and a coffee can. She specializes in writing about family, relationships, cats, psychology and health.

Mesa Foard is a freelance writer in Lexington, South Carolina. Her website is located at *www.mesafoard.com.* She is currently working on her first novel.

Louise Foerster is founder and principal of OpeningDialogue, which provides comprehensive writing services, and of Copper Beech Homeowner Referrals, guiding homeowners to reliable home services. She lives with her family in Darien, Connecticut and enjoys golf, reading, and writing about flying pigs and spa goats.

Pat Gallant's work has appeared in publications such as the *Saturday Evening Post, Writer's Digest, The New Press Literary Quarterly,* and *Chicken Soup for the Writer's Soul.* Her most recent nonfiction can be found in *Family Gatherings, The Simple Pleasures of Friendship,* and *Things That Go Bump in the Night,* three anthologies just published in late 2003 and in 2004. A finalist in the 1991 PEN Syndicated Fiction Project, Pat won the New Century Writer's Award in 1999, 2001, 2002, and 2003, and has been a finalist for the grand prize in the William Faulkner Literary Competition for the last nine years. She has just completed her first book of literary nonfiction shorts, *Holding On to Right-Side Up.* Contact Pat Gallant at *writinggallant@webtv.net, www.PatGallant.com.*

Jennie Ivey lives in Cookeville, Tennessee. She is a newspaper columnist, the author of several fiction and nonfiction stories and co-authored *Tennessee Tales the Textbooks Don't Tell,* a collection of true stories from Tennessee history. This is her third published *Chicken Soup* story. You can contact her at *jivey@frontiernet.net.*

Abha Iyengar has contributed to "The Simple Touch of Fate", "Knit Lit Too", "Science, Technology and Development" and other print anthologies. She is a Kota Press Poetry Anthology Contest winner. Her work has appeared in Insolent Rudder, Raven Chronicles, Gowanus Books, Tatoo Highway, 3 Tryst and Surface Onlline, among others.

Sally Kelly-Engeman is a freelance writer who's had numerous articles and short stories published. In addition to reading, writing and researching, she enjoys ballroom dancing and traveling. She recently returned from an enchanting trip around the world with her husband. She can be reached at *sallyfk@juno.com.*

Candy Killion is a freelance writer whose credits include *America's Intercultural Magazine* and Viva Voce Press' *"They Lied!"* humor anthology; she is also slated to appear in the *Rocking Chair Reader, Cup of Comfort for Love* and *Haunted Encounters* book series in 2005.

Marian Van Eyk McCain is a retired psychotherapist, book reviewer, editor and freelance writer. Her first book, *Transformation through Menopause* (Bergin & Garvey), was described by several reviewers as the best ever written on the pschological and spiritual aspects of menopause. It was followed by *ELDERWOMAN: Reap the wisdom, feel the power, embrace the joy* (Findhorn Press), an inspiration 'trail guide' for the third age journey, and *The Lilypad List: 7 steps to the simple life* (Findhorn Press). Contact Marian through her Web site at *www.elderwoman.org.*

Jacqueline J. Michels is currently enjoying her midlife crisis and has finally decided what she is going to be when she grows up—therefore, she is returning to college to seek her degree in journalism and photography. She is a mother of five and an expectant grandmother.

Jann Mitchell is the author of two books: *Organized Serenity* (1992) and *Codependent for Sure! An Original Joke Book* (1992) as well as a frequent contributor to the *Chicken Soup for the Soul* series. She divides her time between the U.S., Sweden and Tanzania, where she sponsors an African preschool and AIDS orphans. Reach her at *jannmitchell@aol.com.*

Kimberly A. Porrazzo is a senior writer for *OC METRO Magazine* and an award-winning columnist. This is her second *Chicken Soup for the Soul* essay accepted for publication. She is the author of The Nanny Kit (Viking Penguin). Kimberly is married with two teenage sons. Contact her at: *kimberlyporrazzo@cox.net.*

Ferida Wolff is a contributor to *Chicken Soup for the Soul of America, Chicken Soup's Life Lessons for the Woman's Soul,* and *Chocolate For a Teen's Dream.* She is the author of *Listening Outside Listening Inside* and *The Adventures of Swamp Woman,* as well as 14 published books for children. Ferida has been published in *The New York Times, The Philadelphia Inquirer,* national magazines, and poetry journals.

Just what the doctor ordered...

Look for these great topics in the
Chicken Soup for the Soul® Healthy Living Series

Arthritis
Asthma
Breast Cancer
Depression
Diabetes
Heart Disease
Menopause
Pain Management
Stress
Weight Loss

FROM **TOP** MEDICAL EXPERTS!